GIVING VOICE TO WHAT WE KNOW
MARGARET NEWMAN'S THEORY OF HEALTH AS EXPANDING CONSCIOUSNESS IN NURSING PRACTICE, RESEARCH, AND EDUCATION

Carol Picard, PhD, RNC
Professor, School of Nursing
University of Massachusetts
Amherst, Massachusetts
Associate Clinical Scientist
Dana-Farber Cancer Institute Cantor Center
Boston, Massachusetts

Dorothy Jones, EdD, RNC, FAAN
Professor, William F. Connell School of Nursing
Boston College
Chestnut Hill, Massachusetts
Senior Nurse Scientist
Massachusetts General Hospital
Boston, Massachusetts

JONES AND BARTLETT PUBLISHERS
Sudbury, Massachusetts
BOSTON   TORONTO   LONDON   SINGAPORE

World Headquarters
Jones and Bartlett
   Publishers
40 Tall Pine Drive
Sudbury, MA 01776
978-443-5000
info@jbpub.com
www.jbpub.com

Jones and Bartlett
   Publishers Canada
2406 Nikanna Road
Mississauga, ON L5C 2W6
CANADA

Jones and Bartlett
   Publishers International
Barb House, Barb Mews
London W6 7PA
UK

Copyright © 2005 by Jones and Bartlett Publishers, Inc.

Cover image © 2001 images 100ltd

Library of Congress Cataloging-in-Publication Data

Giving voice to what we know : Margaret Newman's theory of health as expanding consciousness in nursing practice, research, and education / [edited by] Carol Picard, Dorothy Jones.
   p. ; cm.
Includes bibliographical references and index.
ISBN 0-7637-2572-2 (pbk.)
1. Newman, Margaret A. 2. Nursing—Philosophy. 3. Health—Philosophy. 4. Consciousness.
[DNLM: 1. Newman, Margaret A. 2. Nursing Theory—Nurses' Instruction. 3. Consciousness—Nurses' Instruction. 4. Education, Nursing—Nurses' Instruction. 5. Nursing Care—psychology—Nurses' Instruction. 6. Nursing Research—Nurses' Instruction. 7. Pattern Recognition—Nurses' Instruction. WY 86 G539 2004] I. Picard, Carol. II. Jones, Dorothy A.
   RT84.5.N4789G545 2004
   610.73'01—dc22

                                                                    2004005544

Production Credits
Acquistions Editor: Kevin Sullivan
Production Manager: Amy Rose
Associate Production Editor: Renée Sekerak
Editorial Assistant: Amy Sibley
Marketing Manager: Ed McKenna
Manufacturing and Inventory Coordinator: Amy Bacus
Composition: Northeast Compositors
Cover Design: Kristin E. Ohlin
Printing and Binding: Malloy, Inc.
Cover Printing: Malloy, Inc.

Printed in the United States of America
08 07 06 05 04   10 9 8 7 6 5 4 3 2 1

We would like to dedicate this book to Dr. Margaret Newman, her friendship, and her commitment to the advancement of nursing science through knowledge development.

Carol Picard and Dorothy Jones

CONTENTS

FOREWORD   xiii

CONTRIBUTORS   xvii

ACKNOWLEDGMENTS   xxi

PREFACE   xxiii

PART ONE   SETTING THE CONTEXT

1   CARING IN THE HUMAN HEALTH EXPERIENCE   3
        Margaret A. Newman
          HEC   4
          Caring and Health   6
          Theory ResearchPractice   8
          Conclusions   9

2   HEALTH AS EXPANDING CONSCIOUSNESS: KNOWLEDGE IN
        THE DISCIPLINE   11
        Carol Picard and Dorothy Jones
          Introduction   11
          Newman and Health as Expanding Consciousness   11
          Praxis   13
          Pattern: Person–Environment Connection   14
          Disorganzation and Disruption as Opportunities for Growth   15
          Nursing Partnership, Insight, and Potential for Action   16
          Uncovering Family Patterns: Movement and Choice   17
          Researcher's Experience: Dialogue as Mutual Process   18
          Capturing Cultural Uniqueness and HEC   18

HEC–Based Models of Practice   19
HEC and Nursing Education   20
Summary   22
Conclusions   24

3   LINKING NEWMAN'S THEORY OF HEALTH AS EXPANDING
         CONSCIOUSNESS TO ETHICS AND CARING   27
Carolyn Hayes
         Introduction   27
         The Nature of Person and the Ethic of Care   27
         Framing the Clinical Dialogue: Ethical Approaches   28
         HEC and Ethics   30
         Nursing's Relational Covenant, Care, and Ethics   31
         Resolving Ethical Issues   34
         Ethics Within HEC Praxis   34
         Exemplar   37

PART TWO   CARING PRAXIS

4   SUFFERING, GROWTH AND POSSIBILITY: HEALTH AS EXPANDING
         CONSCIOUSNESS IN END-OF-LIFE CARE   43
Anne-Marie Barron
         Introduction   43
         A Professional Narrative   43
         Relevant HEC Concepts   45
         Research Methodology   45
         Findings   46
         Exemplar: Carol   47
         Exemplar of Researcher–Staff Connection   49
         Informing Clinical Practice and HEC   50

5   CREATING A HEALING ENVIRONMENT FOR STAFF AND PATIENTS
         IN A PRE–SURGERY CLINIC   53
Jane Flanagan
         Introduction   53
         The Preadmission Nursing Practice Model   53
         The Environment of Care: Beginnings   54
         The Process of Model Development and Implementation   55
         Exemplars of Changed Practice   60
         Conclusions   63

6   THE THEORY IS THE PRACTICE: AN EXEMPLAR   65

Virginia A. Capasso

Nurse Work   65

Exemplar   66

Health as Expanding Consciousness   68

Analysis of the Exemplar   69

Implications   70

Summary   71

7   NURSING PRAXIS OF FAMILY HEALTH   73

Merian Litchfield

Introduction   73

Nursing Praxis   73

Exemplar   74

Praxis Methodology   78

Family Health   81

Conclusion   82

8   ENGAGING WITH COMMUNITIES IN A PATTERN RECOGNITION PROCESS   83

Margaret Dexheimer Pharris

Introduction   83

Relevant HEC Concepts and Community Process   83

HEC: The Unitary Paradigm and Praxis   85

The Pattern Recognition Process for Adolescents   86

The Emerging Pattern of the Community   88

Identifying Barriers to Health for Women and Girls
  of Color   90

Conclusion   93

9   CREATING BALANCE: RHYTHMS AND PATTERNS IN PEOPLE WITH
         DEMENTIA LIVING IN A NURSING HOME   95

Susan Ruka

Introduction   95

HEC and Creating the Environmental Model of Care   96

Dementia and the Family   97

The Model   97

The Care Model for a Nursing Home   100

Rhythm of Care: Synchrony   102

A Work in Progress   104

10   CREATING AN ENVIRONMENT OF CARE IN CLINICAL PRACTICE:
ADMINISTRATIVE AND PRACTICE PERSPECTIVES   105

Amanda Coakley and Edward Coakley

Introduction   105
Care Environments and Nursing Administration   105
Nursing Administrators and Nursing Theory   107
Challenges for Nurse Administrators to Advance Practice   107
Creating Practice Models   108
Developing Theory–Based Practice: An Exemplar   109
Summary   114

PART THREE   RESEARCH AS PRAXIS

11   CREATIVE MOVEMENT AND REFLECTIVE ART: MODES OF
EXPRESSION FOR PARTICIPANT AND RESEARCHER   119

Carol Picard

Introduction   119
Relevant HEC Concepts   119
Creative Movement   120
Reflective Art   121
Research Design Using Creative Movement and Art   122
Findings   123
Discussion   129
Conclusions   130

12   PARENTS OF PERSONS WITH BIPOLAR DISORDER AND
PATTERN RECOGNITION   133

Carol Picard

Introduction   133
Relevant HEC Concepts   134
Literature Review   134
Study Design   135
Findings   136
Research Process and Reflection on Pattern   138
Discussion   139
Conclusions   140

13   CREATING ACTION RESEARCH TEAMS: A PRAXIS MODEL OF CARE   143
Emiko Endo, Hideko Minegishi, and Satsuki Kubo

Introduction   143
Praxis Model of Care   143
Links to HEC   150
Ethical Dimensions of the Project   150
Conclusions   151

14   RECOGNIZING PATTERNS IN THE LIVES OF WOMEN WITH
MULTIPLE SCLEROSIS   153
Jane Neill

Introduction   153
Relevant HEC Concepts   154
Multiple Sclerosis   154
People Living with MS   155
The Women in This Study   156
Pattern Recognition Process   157
Life Patterns of Women Living with MS   157
Underlying Pattern Representations   157
The Women's Stories: Life Patterns, Underlying Patterns, and HEC   159
Health as Expanding Consciousness   161
Photographs Reflecting Pattern and Expanding Consciousness   162
Conclusions   163

PART FOUR   EDUCATION

15   PRAXIS AS A MIRRORING PROCESS: TEACHING PSYCHIATRIC
NURSING GROUNDED IN NEWMAN'S HEALTH AS
EXPANDING CONSCIOUSNESS   169
Carol Picard and Tara Mariolis

Introduction   169
A Caring and Learning Model for Clients and Students:
   Mirroring Praxis   170
A Model of Praxis   171
Expanding Imaginal Margins: Pattern Appreciation   174
Environment and Meaning: The College Campus   175
Appreciating Client's Pattern   176

Appreciating Student's Own Pattern   176
Conclusion   177

16 CULTIVATING A WAY TO SENSE PATTERN WITH ADVANCED
PRACTICE NURSING STUDENTS   179
Hollie Noveletsky–Rosenthal and Kathleen Solomon
Introduction   179
Professional Identity and HEC   179
Structured Reflection   181
Reflection as Process   183
Discussion   184
Integration of Reflective Practice into Advanced
Nursing Practice Curriculum   185
Conclusions   186

17 DOCTORAL STUDENT EXEMPLAR: TRANSFORMATION IN THE
PATIENT–NURSE DYAD   187
Susan M. Lee
Introduction   187
A Critical Care Exemplar: Transformation of the
Patient–Nurse Dyad   187
Paradigmatic Perspectives   189
Linking Theory to Practice   190
The Dynamics of Care   192
Care Practice: Healing, Not Curing   196
Discussion   197
Recommendations for Education: Personal Transformation   199

PART FIVE   DIALOGUE AND COMMENTARY

18 CONVERGENCE AND DIVERGENCE: DIALOGUE OF NURSE THEORISTS:
NEWMAN, WATSON, AND ROY   205
Carol Picard and Dorothy Jones
Introduction   205

19 DIALOGUE OF NEWMAN SCHOLARS AND OTHERS INTERESTED IN HEC   213
Katherine Rosa
Introduction   213
Dialogue and Commentary   213
HEC: Nursing Education and Practice   214
Nursing Knowledge and Art   215

Nursing Knowledge, Philosophy, Intentionality, and Presence   216
Personal Reflection   217
Closing   217

20   CONCLUDING THOUGHTS AND FUTURE DIRECTIONS   219
Dorothy Jones
Theory, Practice, Research: An Iterative Process   220
HEC: Future Directions   224
HEC: Future Considerations   224
Final Thoughts   227

INDEX   229

FOREWORD

MARGARET A. NEWMAN

Dottie Jones once assured me that the theory of health as expanding consciousness (HEC) has a life of its own. This book is a testimony to that life. Its title, *Giving Voice to What We Know*, reveals the relevance of the theory to the unarticulated essence of nursing: the experience of a caring, knowing presence in health as a transformative process.

In my senior year as an undergraduate student in nursing I discovered Dorothy Johnson's (1961) groundbreaking article, "The Significance of Nursing Care," in which she declared that the knowledge of nursing was distinct from the knowledge of medicine. Up to that point, most of what had been taught in the nursing curriculum was about medicine, with a short addendum regarding nursing. Johnson began to explicate the different kind of knowledge needed to practice nursing; she opened the door to the substance of the discipline. Her assertion served the impetus for my entire career in nursing: the development of nursing knowledge. I was encouraged along the way by sensitive mentors to take note of my experiences in nursing, and in 1967 I was drawn to study with Martha Rogers, whose conceptualization of nursing was consistent with my own experiences. Rogers (1970) took the development of nursing knowledge a step further by demanding a shift in paradigm to a focus on a unitary view of the client–environment relationship.

Rogers's view compelled the development of a new concept of health. I struggled with the then popular view of health as existing on a continuum, but ultimately was able to see that acceptance of the continuum perpetuated a dichotomy of health and illness. Recognizing the unitary nature of rhythmic phenomena and convinced by Bentov's (1978) assertion of life as the process of expanding consciousness, I was struck with the revelation of health as *encompassing* disease and as unfolding as expanding consciousness! This realization required an about-face. The futility of always trying to make people well, or prevent their getting sick, was transcended by this concept of health. Nurses could embrace this unitary perspective and enter into meaningful, transformative relationships with their clients regardless of each client's position on the health–illness continuum.

This book presents astounding evidence of how nurses who embrace health as expanding consciousness are contributing to the significance of nursing care. The research focuses on the nurse–client relationship in the process of identifying the clients' unfolding patterns. The theory has no boundaries; it is relevant across cultures and throughout the entire spectrum of health concerns. There are, of course, variations in interpretation of the theory as seen through the lens of each nurse researcher/clinician/author. The interpenetration of the patterns of those involved manifests unique patterns. The variations nevertheless illustrate the unitary, transformative nature of the theory.

Nursing research about HEC incorporates theory, research, and practice in which both the nurse and the client are fully engaged. Not only has HEC made a difference in the lives of the participant clients, but it has also affected the lives of the nurses, who themselves are transformed. In Chapter 5, Jane Flanagan points out that the change is an inner awareness that at times is experienced as an unaccustomed vulnerability as the nurses see themselves in a new way and, despite the uncertainty, find new freedom to truly be a nurse. She adds that once changes consistent with HEC are made, there is "no returning to the previous way care was delivered."

The process often becomes increasingly chaotic and unpredictable as it reaches a turning point. The shared task of the nurse and the client is to "hang in there" until a new direction and pattern are manifest. A number of authors in this book attest to the initial difficulty experienced by nurses as they attempt to stay with this uncertainty. When they are finally able to stand in the center of the chaos, however, the light appears and they experience the exuberance of the transformation. The circumstantial uncertainty is superceded by the inner certainty of the evolution of consciousness to a higher dimension. As several nurses have pointed out, one does not practice nursing *using* the theory, but rather the theory becomes a way of being with the client—a way of offering clients an opportunity to know and be known and to find their way. The nurse's experience resonates with the client's experience and releases transforming energy. The insight gained reveals a path of action.

The theory of health as expanding consciousness emerged from a Rogerian perspective. It connects with theories of caring, and fulfills the commitment of the nursing profession to caring in the human health experience. Dorothy Jones's keen sensitivity to the meaning of the theory is a continuing lighthouse for students and colleagues alike. Carol Picard's creative energy has helped make it possible for these HEC scholars to present their experiences together as evidence of the transformative nature of nursing practice and as a stimulus for further elaboration. I rejoice in the contribution this book makes to the significance of nursing care.

References

Bentov, I. (1978). *Stalking the wild pendulum.* New York, NY: E. P. Dutton.

Johnson, D. E. (1961). The significance of nursing care. *American Journal of Nursing,* 61(11), 63–66.

Rogers, M. E. (1970). *An introduction to the theoretical basis of nursing.* Philadelphia, PA: Davis.

CONTRIBUTORS

Anne-Marie Barron, PhD, APRN-BC
Assistant Professor, Simmons College
Boston, Massachusetts
Clinical Specialist
Massachusetts General Hospital
Boston, Massachusetts

Virginia A. Capasso, Ph.D., APRN-BC
Clinical Specialist, Center for Clinical and Professional Development
Co-Director, Wound Care Center
Massachusetts General Hospital
Assistant Clinical Professor
MGH Institute of Health Professions
Instructor
Harvard Medical School
Boston, Massachusetts

Amanda B. Coakley, Ph.D., R.N.
Staff Specialist
Massachusetts General Hospital
Boston, Massachusetts

Edward Coakley, M.S., R.N.
Deputy Vice-President of Nursing Emeritus
Massachusetts General Hospital
Boston, Massachusetts

Emiko Endo, Ph.D., R.N.
Professor
Miyazaki Prefecture Nursing University
Manabino, Miyazaki, Japan

Jane Flanagan, Ph.D., R.N., APRN-BC
Assistant Professor
University of Massachusetts–Lowell
Lowell, Massachusetts
Associate Clinical Scientist
Dana-Farber Cancer Institute Cantor Center
Boston, Massachusetts

Carolyn Hayes, PhD, RN
Director, Clinical Initiatives
Nursing and Patient Care Services
Dana Farber Cancer Institute
Boston, Massachusetts

Dorothy Jones, EdD, RNC, FAAN
Professor, William F. Connell School of Nursing
Boston College
Chestnut Hill, Massachusetts
Senior Nurse Scientist
Massachusetts General Hospital
Boston, Massachusetts

Satsuki Kubo, PhD, RN
Lecturer, School of Nursing
Kitasato University
Kitasato, Japan

Susan M. Lee, PhD (Candidate), RN, FNP
Doctoral (Candidate), William F. Connell School of Nursing
Boston College
Chestnut Hill, Massachusetts

Merian Litchfield, PhD, RN
Research/Consultant
Wellington, New Zealand

Tara Mariolis, RN, MS, CS
Clinical Instructor
Fitchburg State College
Fitchburg, Massachusetts

Hideko Minegishi, PhD, RN
Associate Professor, School of Nursing
Kitasato University
Kitasato, Japan

Jane Neill, PhD, RN
Senior Lecturer in Nursing, School of Nursing and Midwifery
Flinders University
Adelaide, Australia

Margaret A. Newman, PhD, RN, FAAN
Professor Emeritus
University of Minnesota
Minneapolis, Minnesota

Hollie Noveletsky–Rosenthal, PhD, APRN-BC
Geropsychiatric Nurse Practitioner
York, Maine

Margaret Dexheimer Pharris, PhD, RN, MPH, FAAN
Assistant Professor, Department of Nursing
College of St. Catherine
Minneapolis, Minnesota

Carol Picard, PhD, RNC
Professor, School of Nursing
University of Massachusetts
Amherst, Massachusetts
Associate Clinical Scientist
Dana-Farber Cancer Institute Cantor Center
Boston, Massachusetts

Katherine Rosa, PhD, RN
Assistant Professor
University of Massachusetts
Lowell, Massachusetts

Sr. Callista Roy, PhD, RN, FAAN
Professor and Nurse Theorist, William F. Connell School of Nursing
Boston College
Chestnut Hill, Massachusetts

Susan Ruka, PhD, RN
Nursing Home Administrator
Merriman House
North Conway, New Hampshire

Kathleen Solomon, RN, MS, APRN-BC
Assistant Clinical Professor
MGH Institute of Health Professions
Boston, Massachusetts

Jean Watson, PhD, RN, HNC, FAAN
Distinguished Professor of Nursing
Chair in Caring Sciences
University of Colorado Health Science Center
Denver, Colorado

Acknowledgments

I would like to acknowledge the contributions of doctoral and masters students at Boston College, William F. Connell School of Nursing who have studied the work of Dr. Margaret Newman with me and have advanced nursing science through the application of health as expanding consciousness in research and clinical practice. I would also like to thank my family who have given us the support and love to experience professional nursing and all its potential.

Dorothy A. Jones EdD, RNC, FAAN

Thanks to my family, especially Denis, Alison, and Jeff who have been sources of support and encouragement, and to my parents for their love and encouragement.

Carol Picard PhD, RNC

PREFACE

There are only a few books specifically designed to link a theoretical perspective with nursing knowledge development, clinical practice, education and curriculum development, research, and nursing administration. *Giving Voice to What We Know* has been developed with that goal in mind. At a time when nurses are being asked to justify their contributions to clinical practice outcomes, Margaret Newman's theoretical perspective offers nurses a way to clearly articulate their contributions to both immediate and long-term changes in health. Within the context of a partnership, nurses intentionally engage with the patient and his or her family, to know the person, facilitate choice, promote growth, and uncover meaning about the lived human experience in health and illness. It is the authors' intention to provide new insights into the application of the theory of health as expanding consciousness (HEC) and, in so doing, offer nurses a way to describe dimensions of care that are responsive to partnership, nursing knowledge, and the creative application of that knowledge to reshape health care and the patient care environments. This book is written by nurses who teach, research, and practice within the theoretical framework of HEC. The authors believe that it will serve as a guide for health care system changes to become a framework for nursing education and clinical research, and an important theoretical perspective to influence leaders in healthcare organizations to optimize professional nursing practice and enhance patient- and family-centered care.

Part One of the book provides an overview of HEC. In *Chapter* 1, Margaret Newman offers her most recent thinking about the concept of caring within the context of the human health experience. The chapter reinforces basic theoretical assumptions found in HEC and expands the concept of caring within this framework. Findings from extant research and published reports on practice models and educational innovations are presented and discussed in *Chapter* 2. This overview expands upon these developments and the potential impact of nursing knowledge associated with use of HEC in education, research, and clinical practice. *Chapter* 3 provides a unique addition to the discussion of HEC and its relationship to ethics and patient care. It links the ethics of care and Newman's focus on partnership within the nurse–patient relationship, to anchor disciplinary values and beliefs on the nature of the person, the individual's rights and freedoms, choice, and mutual respect.

In Part Two, HEC serves as a framework to present selected models and exemplars of practice that have been developed and studied by the authors that apply Newman's theoretical perspective in a variety of clinical situations. *Chapter* 4 examines the use of a praxis model and care for persons at the end of life. The model that emerges from the authors' research is described as it is currently being used in an oncology practice. In *Chapter* 5, the reader is introduced to the development and evaluation of a healing environment that transforms physical surroundings within a clinical setting for nurses, patients, and their families. The model intentionally uses nursing knowledge—and HEC in particular—to design a meaning-centered experience for patients visiting a pre-surgery clinic. Findings from research help to illustrate changes in patients and nurses and to reflect the importance of the partnership between the nurse and the patient and the reciprocal effects of that partnership on personal knowing and transformation.

Chapter 6 presents a practice exemplar that illustrates the use of HEC in a home care situation and reflects on dramatic changes in caregiving when the nurse is able to shift the paradigm of care to one of knowing presence. Through attention and inviting the telling of the patient's story, the author relates the effects of disclosure of another "wound" on accelerated wound healing. The results of the encounter support the value of partnership and foster a recognition of the pattern of the whole during pattern appraisal and care delivery.

A praxis model of family care, with its emphasis on partnership is presented in *Chapter* 7. In this discussion, dialogue and mutual reflection offer the family an opportunity for insight and change in their pattern of responding to a complex situation involving a child who has severe asthma. The chapter addresses the importance of partnership not only with the patient but also with the family, and it speaks to the value of reflection within the context of the dialogue. *Chapter* 8 shifts the lens to view wholeness and pattern within community relationships. Two different community problems—namely, violent victimization and barriers to health for women of color—are discussed. The reader has the opportunity to reflect on personal patterns of interaction in the community, as the author presents the intersection of relationship opportunities within the patterns of young men incarcerated for murder and their families, community leaders, and professionals.

Patients with dementia are the focus of *Chapter* 9. In an effort to cope with the challenges of patients who are unable to articulate what is most meaningful for them, the author discusses the creation of an innovative care model in a nursing home. The staff collaborates with families and other caregivers to understand the rhythm of each patient's expressions and create a care model that promotes comfort and a sense of connection. *Chapter* 10 summarizes the challenges of nursing administration and the use of HEC as a vehicle for introducing changes in practice. The authors invite readers to consider evaluating theory-based practice in terms of contributions and impact that nursing science can have on patient care and personal development.

Part Three focuses on research that has used HEC as a praxis methodology to study health with selected groups of participants. In *Chapter* 11, creative movement and reflective art are studied as modes of expression, used to enhance the process of dialogue and pattern recognition in women. *Chapter* 12 illustrates the use of research as praxis with parents of persons with bipolar disorder. The praxis model presented in *Chapter* 13 uses action research with a team of staff nurses, unit leaders, and researchers to creatively bring a HEC-based model of care to the clinical setting. *Chapter* 14 examines the long-term relationships with participants within the HEC praxis methodology and adds photography to promote reflection and uncover meaning in women diagnosed with multiple sclerosis.

Teaching, learning, and nursing education as they relate to HEC are the focus of Part Four. Here processes and strategies are intentionally introduced into the curriculum, and students and faculty actively participate in dialogue and reflection in various courses across levels of study in nursing. *Chapter* 15 reports a meaning-based clinical experience for baccalaureate students and a group of psychiatric clients. Issues associated with promoting quality of care and the importance of the clinical environment are examined within the HEC framework. The use of a mentoring model called a "mirroring process" optimizes faculty presence to support students' presence to the clients. This model fosters partnership between the faculty member, student, and patient in a clinical setting that can be challenging for the learner. In *Chapter* 16, the authors describe a model of reflective practice grounded in HEC for use with advanced practice nursing students. They suggest that reflection is a useful teaching strategy to promote personal growth, connection, and improved clinical learning. In *Chapter* 17, a doctoral student relates classroom learning and a clinical application of HEC. The author links theoretical knowledge within HEC with the presentation of an acute clinical experience in an ICU. Knowledge based on HEC, intentional presence, and caring are used to describe the patient–nurse interaction over several days. Personal reflection, making the linkages between knowledge and practice, and recognizing personal transformation when practicing in HEC are discussed as new knowledge is gained from this experience.

Part Five is devoted to dialogue. A discussion with three leading nursing theorists— Dr. Margaret Newman, Sister Callista Roy, and Dr. Jean Watson— occurred at a planned meeting in Boston. The group was asked by this book's co-authors to focus on whether nursing knowledge development was moving toward theoretical convergence. A transcript of the ensuing dialogue appears in *Chapter* 18. In addition, a meeting of Newman Scholars that occurred following an international nursing conference is presented in *Chapter* 19. This presentation focuses on a synthesis of emerging themes reflected in the discussion of HEC by an international community of scholars familiar in varying degrees with this theory. The book concludes with *Chapter* 20, which summarizes the reflections on the theoretical perspectives and assumptions embedded in HEC, the theory's utility in clinical practice, and its effectiveness as methodology for research. In addition, this chapter offers suggestions for consideration of HEC as a theory that embodies the essence of nursing and a model to generate nursing knowledge, as a teaching strategy, and as a methodology for understanding the human experience in health and illness for the learner, nurse, and care recipient.

PART ONE

SETTING THE CONTEXT

Chapter One

Caring in the Human Health Experience

Margaret A. Newman

How did I become involved in the concept of caring? The focus of my work has been on the meaning of health; yet in answering the essential questions of the discipline, I had to address the nature of the nurse–patient relationship (Newman, 1990). The research of Joanne Butrin (1990, 1992) brought my attention to the concept of caring as a critical factor in the effectiveness of nurse–patient relationships. Butrin's theoretical background was based largely in health as expanding consciousness (HEC), but she did not set out to address this theory. Instead, she conducted an open-ended qualitative study of nurse–patient relationships in which the members of the dyads came from different cultures. Butrin had no presuppositions about what the data would reveal. During the course of her research, characteristics of effective relationships emerged as being mutual expression of positive regard, mutual respect, and mutual understanding. These characteristics were strikingly congruent with the characteristics of caring. When Butrin explored some of the literature on caring, she found similarities between how Watson (1985) described transpersonal caring and how I (Newman, 1986) characterized the nurse–client relationship in HEC. Watson spoke of the relationship as having "the ability to expand . . . human capacities" (1985, p. 59). I spoke of the relationship as moving to "higher levels of consciousness" (Newman, 1986, p. 89). Watson spoke of the ideal of intersubjectivity, in which both persons are involved. I spoke of the nurse and patient as "experiencing the pattern of consciousness formed by their interaction" (Newman, 1986, p. 89). Even when Butrin and I were not looking for it, caring appeared as an important aspect of effective nursing. I know that this revelation comes as no surprise to readers of this book, but this confrontation with data led to my initial realization of the centrality of caring in the nursing process.

Reprinted with permission from the *International Journal for Human Caring*, 6(2), 2002. Copyright 2002 by International Association for Human Caring.

At the same time, faculty colleagues and I were asking ourselves, "What is the focus of the discipline?" We all were examining various views of health and naturally saw health as the central concept of nursing. It was difficult—and for some impossible—to move beyond health as the focus of the discipline. It was clear to others that we could not ignore caring. As we began to explore the literature, we could see that caring theorists held to caring as the essence of nursing. With the question of the focus of the discipline in mind, we saw clearly two central factors. In nursing, health and caring are inextricably linked: One encompasses the other. And so the synthesis of the two concepts, caring in the human health experience, emerged as the true crux of the nursing discipline (Newman, Sime & Corcoran-Perry, 1991). Since then, others have endorsed the uniqueness of this focus. For example, Smith wrote, "No other discipline is developing knowledge related to how this quality of relationship [caring] facilitates health" (1999, p. 19).

Caring in the human health experience is a unitary phenomenon, one of undivided wholeness and transformation. One concept without the other is not sufficient. As readers know, many organizations lay claim to caring, and clearly nurses are not the only group of practitioners to lay claim to health. It is the synthesis of caring and health that provides the focus of the discipline, the mission of the nursing profession. In the realization of the blending of the two concepts, it becomes apparent that nurses who perform tasks of their practice without caring are not practicing nursing. At the same time, the concept of health that one embraces is equally important; it determines what nurses seek in their practice. Is it a concept of health defined by medicine or one that is unique to nursing?

HEC

The concept of HEC (Newman, 1979, 1986, 1994) has emerged from a nursing paradigm introduced by Rogers (1970) and based on (a) a unitary, dynamic view, (b) pattern, as the identifier of wholeness, and (c) transformative unfolding as the process of change. One of the assumptions of HEC is that life is a process of expanding consciousness (Bentov, 1978). Consciousness is a unitary pattern of information that is an inclusive connected-ness with the wholeness of the universe and that affords an infinite repertoire of potential action and an unlimited capacity to love.

This is what health is all about. Health is not separate from disease, as in the medical model. It incorporates disease, when it is present, as pattern of the whole. Persons are not less whole when they are sick (or diseased). The concept of HEC allows nurses to let go of the hopelessness associated with the medical view of many disease conditions and to concentrate on the meaning and power of the evolving process for the person.

Historically, the first step in understanding the process of HEC is to learn to see pattern—to trace its unfolding transformation. Pattern recognition is an essential element in the life process. It is crucial to survival. Skill in pattern recognition protects the hunted from the hunter. It makes it possible for individuals to know when they are compatible and when they are not. Lyahl Watson (1978), a biologist-anthropologist, described a situation among birds when one bird mimicked the song of another bird as a way of getting his attention. The bird didn't sing just any old song; he sang the song of the bird he was calling. By echoing the song of the other bird, he was saying, "I'm talking to you, Buster!" The pattern connects. My earliest research was aimed at seeing what a nurse could accomplish in very short-span relationships with patients (Newman, 1966). It involved connecting with the patient by making a very specific observation about the patient's situation (for example, "You're looking tired"), using the deliberative nursing process described by Orlando (1961). On one occasion the only thing I could come up with was, "Reading the want ads, huh?" That comment opened up a wealth of suppressed concerns of the patient about her physical condition and her future job capabilities, concerns that she had not revealed to any other professional because "they didn't ask me." The comment was personal, specific to the person, and said, "I'm talking to you, Buster!" Compare that to the nurse's common greeting to the patient: "How are you this morning?" The latter interaction is nonspecific and applies to anyone and everyone whom the nurse might contact. But when the nurse comments on something specific to the person, it opens the door to dialogue about the person's situation. More information comes forth, and the pattern evolves from a fuzzy, minimal sketch to something that is recognizable.

In the context of nursing, pattern describes relationships, relationships within the person and relationships with other people and environment. The pattern is a portrayal of the undivided wholeness of all that there is. There are no boundaries. Consciousness, the pattern of the whole that identifies each person, is coextensive in the universe, from rocks to spirit, from animals to humans and beyond (Newman, 1986).

The patterns that people see, hear, and feel (microscopically and macroscopically) show relationships. They involve not just entities, such as hydrogen, but a relationship of entities, like hydrogen to oxygen, as in water, a very different phenomenon from either of its components. They involve not just quantities, like 1, but a relationship of quantities, like 1:2—the beginning of pattern. At a human level, it's not just a qualitative characteristic of a person, like anger, but how the person who is angry relates with others and the environment. Patterns depict relationships. The pattern connects.

In the past, I have said that it is important to understand one's own pattern. That must occur in relation to others. According to H. G. Gadamer, "Only through others do we gain knowledge of ourselves" (as cited in Rabinow & Sullivan, 1979, p. 107). The interpenetration of patterns of two or more persons is the consciousness that allows them to sense into the pattern of the relationship. To experience this pattern fully, one must let go and be totally oneself. If one is open to a full spectrum of consciousness, one is able to enter into a broader spectrum of the client's world. Paying attention to these observable relationships facilitates nurses~ sensing into the underlying pattern, what David Bohm (1980) referred to as the implicate order, which, as I see it, is the ground of consciousness.

The research regarding HEC began with pattern recognition. Having made the assumption that disease is a manifestation of the pattern of the whole, my colleagues and I chose to work with people with various diseases considered to be major health problems. Since then, the research has moved to other health-related situations. Most of the studies concentrated on the process of pattern recognition and the unfolding of expanding consciousness at critical choice points in the participants' lives. In the early studies, an overall pattern that was similar to the disease pattern could be conjectured, but in retrospect, this aspect was not as important in guiding nursing practice as the process that transpired between the nurse and the participant in the transformative unfolding.

The process of pattern recognition focuses on what is meaningful in the lives of the participants. Meaning characterizes pattern. Many people have never really considered what is most meaningful to them. Nurses can elicit stories of what is meaningful and reflect back to the participants the pattern of relationships described in their stories. In this process, the participants experience insight and, with insight, the clarity of the action to be taken. Litchfield (1999) and Endo (1998) have elaborated on the process more fully.

The process leads to insight and action on the part of the client. The client comes to a point in life where the way is not clear. The old rules don't work anymore. The place demands a choice. The nurse is able to support the client during this time of uncertainty as the insight and potential for action are revealed. When the choice is made, the client's life takes an unanticipated direction characterized by greater freedom and connectedness, and more caring relationships, all of which are manifestations of expanding consciousness.

Caring and Health

Gadow (1990) has called for a dialectic of caring and knowing. Pattern recognition, which can be seen as knowing, is a form of caring. The dialectic of caring and knowing unfolds in expanding consciousness, which is revealed in greater caring. The highest level of consciousness is love.

There is a difference between knowledge *about* the participant and knowledge *of the process* of participating ("we" knowledge), which expresses itself as feeling and intuition. Both the professional and the client experience this kind of knowledge. Nursing must engage in a form of knowing that is a mutual process, a knowing from within, not from outside.

Boykin and Schoenhofer (2001), caring theorists, assert that the need, from the standpoint of the patient, is to be known as a person of value. They place caring at a high level of development and emphasize the intention of nursing to nurture "growing in caring" (Boykin & Schoenhofer, 2001, p. 393). The research on HEC started out to be about identifying pattern (knowing) but also yielded data that revealed caring on the parts of the client- participants. For example, in a study with women with breast cancer, participants expressed increasing closeness to others and greater receptivity to others (Moch, 1990). A study with persons with coronary heart disease revealed movement on the part of participants to more meaningful, caring relationships (Newman & Moch, 1991). Finally, an examination of the paradox of expanding consciousness in men who were HIV/AIDS positive revealed an opening up "to a fuller expression of their own caring" (Lamendola & Newman, 1994).

Other researchers working within the context of HEC have seen their practice as a way of actualizing their caring partnerships with clients (Endo, 1998; Jonsdottir, 1995; Kiser-Larson, 1999; Litchfield, 1999; Neill, 2002; Pharris, 2002; Tommet, 1997). Endo and her colleagues (Endo et al., 2000) in Japan see the process of mutuality and pattern recognition (elements of the research protocol associated with HEC) as a caring partnership yielding expressions of caring in the participants as evidence of transformation.

Recently scholars within the Rogerian framework have integrated caring in their descriptions of nursing-science-based approaches to practice: Barrett cited "caring partnerships"; Malinski referred to "knowledgeable caring" (Smith, 1999); and I wrote, "It is time to break with a paradigm of health that focuses on power, manipulation and control and move to one of reflective, compassionate consciousness" (1997, p. 37). And prominent among these syntheses of caring and knowing is the term *caring consciousness*, coined by Watson (1999). In emphasizing the concept of consciousness, Watson cites a number of theorists who endorse a unitary view of consciousness as the ground of all being, a view that I endorse. Other points from Watson's writings on which she and I agree are (a) that nursing is about relation and meaning, (b) that nursing is an integrating (perhaps transforming) force for health care, and (c) that nursing is transcending itself in a framework of expanding consciousness.

There also are differences in the intentions of the two approaches to nursing. Watson seems to be referring to consciousness as an entity that can be used to promote healing. For example, her definition of caring consciousness is "carrying an intentional caring-healing consciousness" (Watson, 1999, p. 10) with a thrust toward truth, beauty, and harmony, whereas I see consciousness as the pattern of the whole, which includes both order and disorder (the ground-of-all-being view). I see the process of evolving to higher consciousness as including disruption and disharmony as well as calm and harmony. Watson talks about making things whole; I assume that things are inherently whole. The difference is that Watson places emphasis on intentional transformation; I rely on the wisdom of the unpredictable unfolding of higher consciousness. I cannot say precisely what these differences mean in terms of the reality of nursing practice. I leave that for others to ponder. I do see the reality of practice as being fully in the present (a present that encompasses past and future), embracing the meaning of the present situation, whatever it may be.

Regardless, the theories of caring and HEC are coming together to define the mission in nursing. Clearly this is not a new path but one that many intuitive practitioners have followed through the years. Theorists have just given it expression in their words. Caring, a form of knowing is transformed into a more inclusive caring at a higher level of consciousness.

TheoryResearchPractice

The neat thing is that the research takes the form of practice! For some nurses schooled in the demands of the scientific method, it has been a winding, uncertain journey from control and predictability to the allowing of the natural phenomenon to express itself in unpredictable ways, but once there, it is clear that the unfolding process reveals expanding consciousness and caring behaviors on the part of the participants. TheoryResearchPractice is a unitary process.

The participants (patients) tell their stories of meaningful events in their lives, and as the pattern of relationships emerges, insight occurs and with it the clarity of potential action. As participants begin to sense the meaning of their own pattern of relationships, they have more confidence in themselves and become more assertive. Transformation will manifest itself in greater freedom, greater connectedness, and more caring relationships.

Is this research scientific? I don't think so, at least not in the usual sense of the word. In the unitary, transformative paradigm, research is defined differently. It is not predictive or repeatable; it is active (applicable) in the moment, it makes a difference (enlightens client about meaning and action potential), and it enlightens the process of practice. It is praxis, which is a mutual process. It is understanding rather than prediction. According to Bernstein (1983), hermeneutics and praxis are the fusion of understanding and application; they are the understanding, interpretation, and application of knowledge. The concept of dialogue is fundamental; it is feeling with. Praxis is more fundamental than method. It is a different genre of research (science?).

In scanning some of the caring literature, I encountered Madeleine Leininger's sunrise model of nursing knowledge discovery (McFarland, 2001) and found it to be fairly consistent with the characteristics of HEC research. The emphasis is on pattern of the whole within a meaningful cultural context. The model focuses on the totality of lifeways of people to grasp a more comprehensive picture of humans in their real life-world (pattern recognition); encourages the researcher or clinician to learn from informants and to let them be in control of ideas (unfolding information that follows the lead of the participant); and may be used in any culture (true for HEC).

If one assumes that each person is a manifestation of one's particular culture and that a nurse is always involved in a transcultural relationship, then can one not say that the approach is culture-free, just as I have said that the approach is disease free? This assertion does not imply that culture and disease are not present but that they are revealed differentially in the pattern portrayal. The approach focuses on the pattern of the whole, wherever and whatever that involves.

Conclusions

In my exploration of caring in the human health experience, I emphasize the dialectic of caring and knowing; I see pattern recognition as the process whereby patients are known; and I see HEC as manifesting itself in caring, connected-ness, insight, and action. The process is specific to each person. The process incorporates the theory and is a form of both practice and research.

The experience of examining the theories of caring and HEC has been one of finding the commonalities of the theories. If there are differences, I think they are in each person's concept of health. From my standpoint, health as pattern of the whole must incorporate the chaos of transformation, knowing that the process ultimately takes one to a more inclusive level of being and connected-ness. The thing that makes a difference in practice is the caring, creative presence of the nurse in recognizing the pattern of the whole.

References

Bentov, I. (1978). *Stalking the wild pendulum*. New York: E. P. Dutton.

Bernstein, R. J. (1983). *Beyond objectivism and relativism: Science, hermeneutics, and praxis*. Philadelphia, PA: University of Pennsylvania.

Bohm, D. (1980). *Wholeness and the implicate order* London, England: Routledge & Kegan Paul.

Boykin, A., & Schoenhofer, S. 0. (2001). Nursing as caring. In M. Parker (Ed.), *Nursing theories and nursing practice* (pp. 391-402). Philadelphia, PA: F. A. Davis.

Butrin, J. E. (1990). The experience of culturally diverse nurse-client encounters (Doctoral dissertation, University of Minnesota, 1990). *Dissertation Abstracts International*, 51(06), 2815B.

Butrin, J. E. (1992). Cultural diversity in the nurse-client encounter. *Clinical Nursing Research*, 1(3), 238–251.

Endo, E. (1998). Pattern recognition as a nursing intervention with Japanese women with ovarian cancer. *Advances in Nursing Science*, 20(4), 49–61.

Endo, E., Nitta, N., Inayoshi, M., Saito, R., Takemura, K., Minegishi, H., Kubo, S., & Kondo, M. (2000). Pattern recognition as a caring partnership in families with cancer. *Journal of Advanced Nursing*, 32(3), 603–610.

Gadow, S. (1990, October). *Beyond dualism: The dialectic of caring and knowing*. Paper presented at the conference on Education for Ethical Nursing Practice, University of Minnesota, Minneapolis.

Jonsdottir, H. (1995). Life patterns of people with chronic obstructive pulmonary disease: Isolation and being closed in (Doctoral dissertation, University of Minnesota, 1995). *Dissertation Abstracts International*, 56(03), 1 346B.

Kiser-Larson, N. (1999). Life patterns of Native American women experiencing breast cancer (Doctoral dissertation, University of Minnesota, 1999). *Dissertation Abstracts International*,60(05), 2062B.

Lamendola, F. P., & Newman, M. A. (1994). The paradox of HIV/AIDS and expanding consciousness. *Advances in Nursing Science*, 16(3), 13–21.

Litchfield, M. (1999). Practice wisdom. *Advances in Nursing Science*, 22(2), 62–73.

McFarland, M. R. (2001). The ethnonursing research method and the culture care theory: Implications for clinical nursing practice. In M. Parker (Ed.), *Nursing theories and nursing practice* (pp. 377–390). Philadelphia, PA: F. A. Davis.

Moch, S. D. (1990). Health within the experience of breast cancer. *Journal of Advanced Nursing*, 15, 1426–1435.

Neill, J. (2002). Transcendence and transformation in the life patterns of women living with rheumatoid arthritis. *Advances in Nursing Science*, 24(4), 27–47.

Newman, M. A. (1966). Identifying patients' needs in short-span nurse-patient relationships. *Nursing Forum*,5(1), 76–86.

Newman, M. A. (1979). *Theory development in nursing*. Philadelphia, PA: F. A. Davis.

Newman, M. A. (1986). *Health as expanding consciousness*. St. Louis, MO: Mosby.

Newman, M. A. (1990). Nursing paradigms and realities. In N. L. Chaska (Ed.), *The nursing profession: Turning points* (pp. 230–235). St. Louis, MO: Mosby.

Newman, M. A. (1994). *Health as expanding consciousness* (2nd ed.). New York, NY: National League for Nursing Press.

Newman, M. A. (1997). Experiencing the whole. *Advances in Nursing Science*,20(1), 34–39.

Newman, M. A. (2002). The pattern that connects. *Advances in Nursing Science*,24(3), 1–7.

Newman, M. A., & Moch, S. D. (1991). Life patterns of persons with coronary heart disease. *Nursing Science Quarterly*, 4(4), 161–167.

Newman, M. A., Sime, A. M., & Corcoran-Perry, S. A. (1991). The focus of the discipline of nursing. *Advances in Nursing Science*, 14(1), 1–6.

Orlando, I. J. (1961). *The dynamic nurse-patient relationship*. New York, NY: Putnam.

Pharris, M. D. (2002). Coming to know ourselves as community through a nursing partnership with adolescents convicted of murder. *Advances in Nursing Science*, 24(3), 21–42.

Rabinow, P., & Sullivan, W. M. (Eds.). (1979). *Interpretive social science: A reader*. Berkeley, CA: University of California Press.

Rogers, M. E. (1970). *An introduction to the theoretical basis of nursing*. Philadelphia: F. A. Davis.

Smith, M. (1999). Caring and the science of unitary human beings. *Advances in Nursing Science*, 21(4), 14–28.

CHAPTER TWO

HEALTH AS EXPANDING CONSCIOUSNESS: KNOWLEDGE IN THE DISCIPLINE

CAROL PICARD

DOROTHY JONES

Introduction

Since Margaret Newman published her initial thinking on the theory of health as expanding consciousness (HEC) in 1979, scholars, educators, and practicing nurses have explored the utility of the theory through their own work. Some have taken the theory and embodied it, while others have used it to ground research, clinical practice, and teaching. This chapter examines knowledge gained from research using Newman's research praxis with a variety of groups differing in terms of their populations, settings, and social experiences. Also in this chapter are reports from nursing leaders engaged in changing practice through dialogue, and educators who challenge students with new ways to study the human experience. Knowledge gained from these investigators will be discussed along with directions for further development and testing of HEC.

Newman and Health as Expanding Consciousness

In Chapter 1, Margaret Newman identified the central concepts and assumptions underlying HEC. Within that discussion, the unitary, undivided, and unfolding nature of pattern of person, the person–environment relationship, and nursing as caring partnership were presented. Knowledge about participants (from without) and knowledge about process (from within the relationship with participants) were described with an emphasis on valuing the caring presence of the nurse and knowing (Newman, 2002).

For Newman, partnership is a deliberative process of engagement both for the clinician and for the researcher. It requires an approach to knowledge development and utilization in nursing that is participatory in nature. Newman challenges nurses to examine their own process of interaction within a relationship. This self-knowledge can enhance the nurse's ability to sense the unfolding pattern in patients, families, and communities. Newman appreciates disease as one manifestation of the overall pattern, and as a manifestation of health. Wholeness, connectedness, and meaning within the lived experience are central to the theory of health as expanding consciousness.

Consciousness is an evolving process. Newman (1990) establishes a parallel between the conceptualization of HEC and Young's (1976) theory of evolution of human movement, depicted as a progression from potential freedom to real freedom, as a conceptual way to explain expanding consciousness. Figure 2.1 illustrates the integration of concepts in Newman's theory and Young's conceptualizations.

The process begins at a point of *potential freedom*. This stage of consciousness precedes the *binding stage* in matter, when we are born. Newman identifies the concept of time with this binding stage of consciousness. In Young's schema, persons are bound when there is no sense of self as individual and decisions are made by others. At the next stage of centering, self-consciousness and identity emerge and the person is focused on self and a reliance on an established order or ways of relating to one's world. Newman identifies the concept of space with this stage, in which a person gains power and some sense of control over others.

Choice is the next phase that emerges in this evolving process. Here the old rules no longer apply, and a need arises to be more reflective in responding to situations. Young describes a *choice point* as a reflective turn in consciousness. Newman believes that this is a turning point, and relates it to the concept of movement. This shift or destabilizing of established order in the choice stage promotes movement and the expansion of consciousness.

The *de-centering stage* occurs once a choice is made, a change in the self takes place, and a movement toward growth and higher levels of freedom continues. Energy at this stage comes from sharing it with others. This idea is related to Newman's concept of boundarylessness, in which a person has the awareness of extending beyond his or her physical boundaries. The unbinding stage occurs as the person is freed from bounds of time and is able to be more fully present in the moment; it correlates with Newman's stage of timelessness. Newman equated Young's stage of real freedom with love and a state of unity in which all opposites are reconciled.

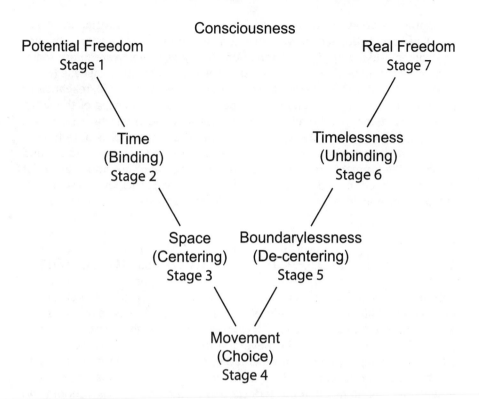

Figure 2.1. Newman's Concepts and Young's Stages of Evolution of Consciousness.
Source: A developing discipline: selected works of Margaret Newman (p. 132) by Margaret A. Newman, 1995, New York: National League for Nursing. Copyright 1995 by Margaret A. Newman. Reprinted with permission.

Praxis

The research method suggested by Newman is one in which the researcher embodies the theory. Praxis, as described by Newman (1990, 1994, 1997, 1999), involves a deep appreciation by the researcher of the nature of expanding consciousness, pattern, and relationship, and the application of that knowledge to dialogue with participants. By inviting research participants to engage in dialogue about the persons and events most meaningful in their lives, the researcher creates an opportunity for reflection, awareness, and potential insight. Some individuals' stories might be expressed in words, whereas others might use aesthetics to express or complement the dialogue. Neill, for example, invited participants with multiple sclerosis to take photographs to express life meanings, as discussed in Chapter 14.

Another strategy used to express meaning relies on movement. Picard (2000) used intentional creative movement as a mode of expression with mid-life women. Ruka employed observation strategies to gain careful appreciation of the meaning of movement for persons with Alzheimer's disease (Ruka, Chapter 9). Using Newman's research method as praxis, the researcher's presence creates an environment for the sharing and receiving of the story. According to Newman, the relationship is central to the unfolding experience. Through dialogue and subsequent reflection, the researcher is able to construct a visual representation of how he or she understands pattern and meaning. Sharing this representation creates yet another opportunity for dialogue, reflection, and pattern recognition by the participants. Visual representations may also be expressed in reflective artwork (Picard, Chapter 12).

Pattern: Person–Environment Connection

Pattern reflects in the expressed value of relationship to others, to self, and to one's spiritual life. The challenges of loss, illness, and threats to relationships were expressed in a study of mid-life women through themes reflecting personal meaning (Picard, 2000). Several studies have described expansion of consciousness as a process in which acceptance and letting go of trying to control one's world can lead to an increased sense of relatedness and movement. This transformation is described by themes such as freedom and peace, being open, self-coherence, or dwelling in a different place (Fryback, 1993; Lamendola & Newman, 1994; Endo, 1998, 2000; Neill, 2002b; Kiser-Larson, 2002).

Serious illness experiences can be associated with a pattern losses of important interpersonal connections early in life. Studies have reported that individuals with long-term illnesses such as cancer (Endo, 1998; Kiser-Larson, 2002; Newman, 1995) and obstructive lung disease (Jonsdottir, 1998; Noveletsky-Rosenthal, 1996) often describe significant losses early in life. Across studies, the experience of feeling disconnected, alone, isolated, or separated from family, loved ones, or community was frequently described as a source of distress within participants' overall pattern.

Smith (1997a, 1997b) explored the nature of person–environment connection with women who had previously experienced sexual victimization. These women reflected a pattern of isolation, lack of positive connections in social relationships with their families, and a high sense of external control. This lack of connectedness was also reported in Pharris's work with adolescents convicted of murder (2002). This study described participants' acts of violence as a last desperate attempt to connect in some way with the community when they felt extremely isolated from everyone. Capasso's exemplar (Chapter 6) with an individual who was experiencing delayed wound healing reports how an early childhood trauma and subsequent problems being connected with others were sources of the patient's continuing distress. Disclosing this information through dialogue seemed to affect choices and new insights for the patient.

All researchers using Newman's praxis methodology report that, for some participants, the research process of dialogue was a person–environment connection that provided a new opportunity to experience pattern recognition. Although few studies have incorporated long-term contact with participants, those with a one-year follow-up have reported individual accounts of change continuing to unfold (Litchfield, 1999; Neill, 2002b; Tommet, 2003; Yamashita, 1999).

Disorganization and Disruption as Opportunities for Growth

Newman (1994) has posited that periods of disorganization and disruption in pattern may act as a catalyst for expansion of consciousness. Illness experiences can be sources of disruption. In several studies, participants with a serious illness have described disruptive periods that were often followed by changes in conscious awareness, or shifts in perspective. Subjects often spoke of being grateful for the new knowledge gained through the experience, such as seeing what is most important in life, valuing and attending to relationships, changing priorities to accommodate what is meaningful, attending to self-care, and finding pleasure in simple things (Moch, 1990; Fryback, 1993; Lamendola & Newman, 1994). According to some researchers, following the diagnosis of a disease process, participants took the opportunity to reflect on their own self-care. Prior to the disruption, their obligations to others often took precedent over basic activities of self-care and restoration. The illness experience provided a wake-up call for choosing wisely and attending to their personal needs (DeMarco, Picard & Agretelis, 2004; Fryback, 1993; Koob, Roux & Bush, 2002; Moch, 1990; Neill, 2002b; Newman, 1995; Picard, 2000; Kiser-Larson, 2002).

Restricted movement associated with an illness or incarceration became an opportunity for inner reflection, similar to the findings in Newman's early work (Moch, 1990; Pharris, 2002; Neill, 2002a; Koob, Roux & Bush, 2002). Jonsdottir's (1998) study, describing persons with chronic obstructive pulmonary disease (COPD), found that the disease's physical demands were part of a pattern of personal isolation and limited person–environment connection. Many participants reported a need to maintain a stable and unchanging life situation to preserve their energy and reduce the strain on their pulmonary status. Jonsdottir also noted the participants' patterns of relating were in some ways reflective of the disease process itself—that is, being "closed in." Noveletsky-Rosenthal (1996) reported a similar pattern for a subgroup of participants also experiencing COPD, who reported isolation and a block in connecting with others and the larger environment.

Karian, Jankowski, and Beal (1998) interviewed adults who were childhood cancer survivors. Participants attributed a change in awareness associated with their illness experiences. This awareness was manifested by an increased connection with others, an empathic response to their world, a desire to help others, and a changed perspective on the value of life and loved ones. Subsequent to the illness, participants reported making decisions more mindfully, with an appreciation of choosing wisely how to spend their time. Moch's (1990) research with cancer survivors generated similar findings. In another study involving nurse cancer survivors, participants reported that following a period of chaos and disruption associated with their illness, they experienced a deepening level of compassion, becoming advocates for creating caring practices, and a reordering of priorities that sought to place relationships to self and others in the forefront (Picard, Agretelis & Demarco, 2004; DeMarco, Picard & Agretelis, 2004).

Smith (1997a, 1997b) and Picard (1998) found some study participants who noted that, following experiences of chaos and disruption in childhood, the most important factor facilitating healing was being part of a single caring relationship as adults. This situation was described as a relationship in which another person (i.e., spouse, friend, grandparent) reached out and accepted the participant unconditionally. Participants associated the transformation in their lives with truly being known for their uniqueness.

Nursing Partnership, Insight, and Potential for Action

When persons are in the midst of a turbulent period, such as during an illness, they may be unable to recognize their own pattern or its underlying meaning. A partnership with a nurse during these periods can create an opportunity for reflection on pattern and a shift in perspective (Jonsdottir, Litchfield & Pharris, 2003). Litchfield's research noted that as families engaged in dialogue with the nurse/researcher, they experienced insight into their pattern, and the illness of their child moved from being a focal point in the family to an integrated aspect of the family's pattern (1999). To integrate is to take something in, rather to look out upon a focal point. Gaining perspective is what Litchfield calls an "expanding horizon" (p. 68). In this study, parents were able to see their family's pattern over time. The insight potential offered through dialogue and pattern recognition allowed each family to move toward fully accepting their pattern and living more fully in the present.

Several researchers have noted that the process of partnership within the research/praxis approach was often experienced by participants as a source of strength and opportunity for insight (Barron, 2002; Endo, 1998, 2000; Pharris, 2002; Picard, 2000; Tommet, 2003). The chance to reflect upon meaning across one's life was viewed as a new opportunity. For example, Tommet reported that when a caring partnership with a nurse existed, participants described making order out of the chaos as coming more easily while caring for their medically fragile child.

Other researchers (Yamashita 1999; Koob, Roux & Bush, 2002; Demarco, Picard & Agretelis, 2004; Picard, Chapter 12; Tommet, 2003) report that the absence of a caring connection with health professionals (nurses) contributed to further distress and added to the challenge of the illness experience. For example, poor communication and a callous manner on the part of health professionals contributed to participants' feelings of suffering alone with the child's mental illness (Yamashita, 1999).

Uncovering Family Patterns: Movement and Choice

Several researchers have used Newman's HEC to explore family patterns. Yamashita (1999) studied the patterns of families in which a member was diagnosed with schizophrenia. This investigation found families experiencing aloneness in the struggle with mental illness. They described a lack of connectedness with professionals, along with limited information to help them understand their family member's behaviors. When families were able to accept the illness, it marked a turning point for the individuals involved. This change was manifested by family members becoming more open, able to disclose their situation to others, and ask for help. When family members were presented with a rendering of their family pattern, they engaged in dialogue with the researcher. The praxis process seemed to provide an opportunity for insight, and the potential for action and change was realized.

Recent work with families of women experiencing ovarian cancer (Endo, 2000) and a family's response to the death of a child (Picard, 2002) indicated that family members regulated their energy and rhythm in response to one another, restricting their expression of sadness to each other regarding painful issues. Once dialogue occurred around the sharing of meaning and acceptance of the situation, changes occurred in the quality of interactions between family members. Family members were also able to see the larger shared family pattern of meaning.

Tommet (2003) and Litchfield (1999) researched the pattern of nurse–parent interactions in families with ill children. In these situations, the nurse–parent relationship served as the vehicle for participant families to find meaning in the chaos of the family–environment pattern as they negotiated and struggled with various aspects of the health care system in seeking resources for their children.

Researcher's Experience: Dialogue as Mutual Process

Researchers using HEC have reported an increased appreciation for their own pattern of interaction and a broader appreciation of patient concerns within their practice, both coming as a result of the research process. Moch (1990) examined the researcher's process in partnership and published a text on the subject (Moch & Gates, 2000). The author used poetry to capture personal feelings about process. Similarly, nurses involved in working with patients in a pre-surgical unit found the research process difficult to put into words and often used art and poetry to articulate what was changing in them because of the process (Flanagan, 2002).

Neill (2002a) described how the caring praxis of the research process changed her concept of nursing as well as gave insights about her own pattern of relationships and meaning. After using a praxis method with patients experiencing advanced cancer, Barron (2001) found that she could not return to the way she had practiced nursing previously. The experience pointed to the mutuality in the HEC-based dialogue. Pharris's (2002) research highlighted the ways in which both individual nurses and communities reflected on their own roles in the lives of troubled adolescent boys. This research invited community members to see themselves as part of the adolescents' environment and to consider dialogue and engagement as vehicles for evolving the health of the community as a whole.

Capturing Cultural Uniqueness and HEC

Only one researcher has reported using a HEC perspective to specifically examine the role of culture and its influence on encounters between nurses and clients. Prior to the development of Newman's protocol, Butrin (1992) interviewed nurses and patients separately to elicit their expectations and satisfaction after a clinical encounter. Findings indicated that despite language differences (using a translator), mutual satisfaction with the nurse–patient dyad interactions occurred when participants experienced respect, a feeling of being understood, and a sense of shared values. The study concluded that ethnocentrism, stereotyping, and language challenges were the main barriers to satisfaction in clinical encounters for both parties, and that cultural differences were not a major factor.

Researchers using Newman's praxis method reported other selected study findings related to culture. Two immigrant families in Yamashita's (1999) study believed that health professionals in their new country engaged in stereotyping. This perceived attitude blocked any meaningful dialogue with those providers. Kiser-Larson (2002) also used Newman's research praxis with Native American women who had breast cancer. These women believed that the poverty and deprivation they experienced were related to discrimination by the dominant culture.

HEC-Based Models of Practice

Early work using practice/praxis was completed by Margaret Newman in conjunction with nurse leaders in two health systems. Newman, Lamb, and Michaels (1991) reported using a case management model of care, consistent with HEC. Newman spent three months with the case management team, using the hermeneutic dialectic process of inquiry with the staff to explore the nature of their practice. During the course of the dialogue and pattern appraisal, pattern recognition began to emerge, along with an appreciation of the nature of timing of interactions and a sense of openness to each person's unfolding process. The nurses in the project understood that an important piece of their work was to support patients' choices and offer knowledge to patients in a nonjudgmental way. With an emphasis on wholeness, choices were seen as opportunities for personal growth.

Bunkers and her colleagues (1992) and Koerner and Bunkers (1994) also invited Newman to consult across several healthcare systems in Sioux Falls, South Dakota. These scholars were among the first to examine the use of HEC as a theoretical basis for grounding a model of integration between practice and education. The authors used the symbol of a spider's web from Navaho creation mythology to illustrate the interconnectedness among the basic values and principles of Newman's theory, organizational structures, and caring practices. As part of this analysis, the caring capacities of the nurse were identified as pattern recognition, sensing into self, creative tension, therapeutic alliance, and disciplined presence.

Research within the clinical setting also contributes to nursing science by articulating the various relationships among people: between nurse and patient, between nurse and nurse, and between nurse and system in caring community. The authors cited above offered nurse leaders the needed ingredients for successful systems development, including a leadership model of mutuality as well as circular and nonhierarchical structures of cross-system interaction through attentive listening and dialogue. When exposed to the process of dialogue, participants came to appreciate the pattern of wholeness and coming together in cooperation. They voiced a commitment to authentic action. In addition, this work demonstrated the use of the HEC protocol within a group format.

Kalb (1990) described a clinical project in which pattern recognition served as the basis for grounding the care of women in preterm labor. A team of nurses and perinatologists helped women to recognize the patterns of fetal movement as a component of the recognition of the pattern of the whole of their pregnancies. Patients self-monitored their need for medication intervention. The team emphasized a care approach looking at the pregnant person as a whole in interaction with the environment. Through a process of dialogue, both the nurses and the pregnant women changed their perspectives on the problem of preterm labor. Kalb reported that although preterm labor was an unwanted element in pregnancy, the women reported that the opportunity to develop an increased awareness of these patterns of interrelationships with the fetus and with their world was a gift.

In another clinical practice model, Schlotzhauer and Farnham (1997) reported a HEC-based school nurse case management practice with children diagnosed with diabetes. Throughout the experience, nurses partnered with students living with diabetes to understand their pattern of energy expenditure in the context of the adolescents' world of school, family, and social relations. Their findings helped nurses gain new insights about the illness experience and helped guide future care with this population.

Work by Flanagan (2002) reflected the use of HEC as an effective strategy to improve patient care in a preadmission clinic. By designing a care model that focused on dialogue, the nurses helped clients use the experience of surgery to uncover pattern and meaning. For many, the experience was life changing. More importantly, the research provided a model for creating a practice environment that promotes healing for both the nurse and the patient.

HEC and Nursing Education

Many undergraduate programs present nursing theory as a topic within a course, but few integrate this content in a meaningful way as part of classroom and clinical learning experience. There has been limited research reported on the use of overall theoretical knowledge to ground and guide nursing education. To fully appreciate the effects of any theory, and of HEC in particular, students must be given opportunities to work with the process over time. As they gain knowledge of theoretical principles and assumptions, they must also have purposeful learning experiences built into the curriculum to demonstrate linkages between theory, practice, and research. In one project, students were invited to share what was most meaningful to them as a way to appreciate their own pattern as well as to experience both presence and dialogue with their clinical faculty and peers (Picard & Mariolis, 2002). This process offered students a way to come to know the theory and to experience its influence in their own lives (Chapter 15).

Jacono and Jacono (1996) grounded their teaching practices by using Newman's HEC as a strategy to cultivate student creativity. Using a reflective process of contemplation for themselves and for students, the authors found that students were able to see a wider array of possibilities for patient–nurse experiences in clinical situations. Their process invited students to use their inner wisdom and insight to take in the full experience between nurse and patient. Again, this mirroring process used by faculty helped student nurses to appreciate the inner wisdom and insight that clients hold about their health/life experiences as well.

Weingourt (1998) worked with nursing students in a nursing home setting to ground clinical practice experiences within a HEC framework. In addition to participating in theory-guided seminars, students discussed both their own and residents' patterns of interaction. Students focused on activities that encouraged person–environment connections and related these experiences to the theoretical underpinnings of HEC. Weingourt encouraged students to control the urge to act, and to first appreciate patterns and meanings expressed by the residents. Students cultivated a way of seeing the disorder and disconnections of patients as part of the pattern of the whole and began to see nursing action as a process instead of a series of goal-driven encounters. Patients expressed less distress and were more peaceful after a series of encounters with these students.

The process of coming to know one's own pattern was also explored with graduate students (Noveletsky-Rosenthal & Solomon, 2001). The authors found that employing a reflective writing process enabled students to sense the pattern of their clinical practice as well as the evolving pattern of self. Seminar dialogue was also described as being beneficial to each student's reflective process. This example helped to model behaviors and experiences that could then be used with patients (Chapter 16).

Doctoral students who were exposed to Newman's research/praxis methodology in a course (Jones, 2003) that provided students with opportunities to use, critique, and evaluate HEC as a way to uncover knowledge and test theory, found the experience to be renewing and exciting. Many described HEC as a way to reconnect with patients at a new level and evaluate responses and the meaning of holistic care in a new way. An exemplar from one student provides thoughtful reflection on the experience and depicts new awareness in the meaning and presence of the nurse in an intentional relationship with the patient (Lee, Chapter 17).

Summary

HEC as Methodology, Guide for Practice, and Framework for Curriculum

Newman's (1994) protocol for research on health as expanding consciousness (pp. 147–149) guides the researcher/clinician and educator to spend time in dialogue with individuals (families and communities) and to focus on meaningful experiences. The goal is a partnership that reflects on the emerging pattern of the whole. Through partnership with the individual, the story is then presented in a visual depiction that represents data segments in chronological order and reflects relationships and events as described by participants during the interview. The process occurs over several interviews, and the pattern that emerges is shared with the participants to validate the story (pattern recognition) and promote reflection.

Whether this praxis method is used to guide clinical practice, focus curriculum and related nursing experiences, or provide a protocol for research, HEC does offer opportunities for creative practice and education models and advancing research and knowledge development within nursing science.

As a Methodology

- HEC is a meaningful process for both the participant and the nurse.
- As a method, it provides the researcher with an opportunity to focus the human experience within the context of a partnership and an embodiment of theory.
- HEC provides a method to understand life experiences within the person's perception of meaning and context.
- Dwelling with the narrative data enables the researcher to reflect pattern as experienced in the dialogue.
- Sharing a pattern display with the participant can promote pattern recognition by the participant and stimulate additional thinking and reflection.
- Looking across patterns as reflected by participants within a study reveals commonalities that can be shaped into testable propositions for further study. This includes information uncovered through HEC-guided research that suggests the following:
  a. Paying attention to the meaning of disconnections and losses in childhood and life choices, events, and relationships
  b. Recognizing the importance of a meaningful relationship and support and initiating and sustaining life changes
  c. Pattern recognition and times of turbulence are opportunities for growth, healing, and transformation
  d. Appreciating that individuals make choices and decisions consistent with learned values and beliefs

e. Making personal discoveries and gaining awareness that can result in behavior change that promotes health, allows for integration of illness into the pattern of the whole, and provides an opportunity for finding meaning in dying

f. Knowing that observation of nonverbal expressions can reveal patterns

g. Use of movement, art, and other forms of aesthetic knowing enhances pattern recognition and clarifies meaning for the participant and the nurse

As a Guide for Creative Practice

- HEC focuses on the person and the nurse in intentional partnership.
- Pattern appraisal allows patients to reflect on what is most important and meaningful in their lives and provides new insights.
- The relationship between the nurse and the participant is central to the caring process.
- HEC fosters the development of an environment of care that promotes knowing the patient and holistic healing.
- Pattern recognition reflects meaning and understanding within the context of life experiences and the recognition of the past as existing in the present with vision for future action.
- The dialogue and intentional presence of the nurse enables pattern appreciation and recognition for the participant and the nurse.
- Pattern recognition creates the potential for insight, awareness, and change.
- Pattern appreciation offers the participant an opportunity to move on and let go of those relationships and events that have created boundaries.
- HEC acknowledges that a nursing model of care can increase the visibility of nursing in promoting sustained behavior change and supportive relationships.
- Illness can be both a time of chaos and an opportunity for change, awareness growth, and integration when nursing care is purposeful and engaging.
- Pattern recognition is integral to choice, movement, transformation, and expanding consciousness.

As a Guide for Education and Curriculum Development

- HEC advances the philosophical values and beliefs consistent with the disciplinary perspective.
- It promotes a nursing ontology that focuses on partnership between nurse and patient (family and community).
- Students at all levels may gain a clearer perspective on nursing's unique identity and contributions to care outcomes.
- The HEC model focuses on process and dialogue as a way to come to know the human experience.
- Pattern appraisal, engagement, and reflection offer a way for a nurse to partner in patient-focused care.
- HEC provides a framework for creating a curriculum that acknowledges the linkages between nursing theory, research, and practice.

- It creates a spirit of inquiry in the learner and enhances knowledge development and research within the nurse–patient experience.
- Faculty can use this approach to model caring behaviors and optimize the contributions of nursing science to national health care, social reform policy change, and global health.

Conclusions

This chapter has presented a summary of research and practice models in education and clinical settings developed by nurses using HEC as a framework. Litchfield (1999) writes that this knowledge merges epistemology (knowledge in and about nursing) and ontology (what nursing is) into practice wisdom. Later chapters in this book present practice models that address the value of bringing the research process into practice and forging partnerships with practicing nurses to create changing health environments with a perspective of wholeness.

References

Barron, A. M. (2001). Life meanings and the experience of cancer. *Dissertation Abstracts International,* 54, 3B (UMI No. 30-08589).

Bunkers, S. (1992). The healing web: A transformation model for nursing. *Nursing and Health Care,* 13(2), 68–73.

Butrin, J. E. (1992). Cultural diversity in the nurse–client encounter. *Clinical Nursing Research,* 1(3), 238–251.

DeMarco, R., Picard, C. & Agretelis, J. (2004). Nurse experiences as cancer survivors: Part I–Personal. *Oncology Nursing Forum,* 31(3), 523–530.

Endo, E. (1998). Pattern recognition as a nursing intervention with Japanese women with ovarian cancer. *Advances in Nursing Science,* 20(4), 49–61.

Endo, E. (2000). Pattern recognition as a caring partnership in families with cancer. *Journal of Advanced Nursing,* 32(3), 603–610.

Flanagan, J. (2002). Nurse and patient perceptions of the pre-admission nursing practice model: Linking theory to practice. *Dissertation Abstracts International* 56 (UMI No. 30-53657).

Fryback, P. B. (1993). Health for people with a terminal diagnosis. *Nursing Science Quarterly,* 6(3), 147–159.

Jacono, B. J., & Jacono, J. J. (1996). The benefits of Newman and Parse in helping nurse teachers determine methods to enhance student creativity. *Nurse Education Today,* 16(5), 356–362.

Jones, D. A. (2003). *Nursing and expanding paradigms* (NU 820). Chestnut Hill, MA: Boston College, William F. Connell School of Nursing.

Jonsdottir, H. (1998). Life patterns of people living with chronic obstructive pulmonary disease: Isolation and being closed in. *Nursing Science Quarterly,* 11(4), 160–166.

Jonsdottir, H., Litchfield, M., & Pharris, M. D. (2003). Partnership in practice. *Research and Theory for Nursing Practice: An International Journal*, 17(1), 51–63.

Kalb, K. A. (1990). The gift: Applying Margaret Newman's theory of health in nursing practice. In M. E. Parker (Ed.), *Nursing theories in practice* (pp. 163–186). New York, NY: National League for Nursing.

Karian, V. E., Jankowski, S. M., & Beal, J. A. (1998). Exploring the lived experience of childhood cancer survivors. *Journal of Pediatric Oncology Nursing*, 15(3), 153–162.

Kiser-Larson, N. (2002). Life pattern of Native American women experiencing breast cancer. *International Journal for Human Caring*, 6(2), 61–68.

Koerner, J. G., & Bunkers, S. S. (1994). The healing web: An expansion of consciousness. *Journal of Holistic Nursing*, 12(1), 51–63.

Koob, P. B., Roux, G., & Bush, H. A. (2002). Inner strength of women dwelling in the world of multiple sclerosis. *International Journal for Human Caring*, 6(2), 20–27.

Lamendola, F., & Newman, M. A. (1994). The paradox of HIV/AIDS as expanding consciousness. *Advances in Nursing Science*, 16(3), 13–21.

Litchfield, M. (1999). Practice wisdom. *Advances in Nursing Science*, 22(2), 62–73.

Moch, S. D. (1990). Health within the experience of breast cancer. *Journal of Advanced Nursing*, 15, 1426–1435.

Moch, S., & Gates, M. (Eds.) (2000). *The researcher experience in qualitative research*. New York, NY: National League for Nursing.

Neill, J. (2002a). From practice to caring praxis through Newman's theory of health as expanding consciousness: A personal journey. *International Journal for Human Caring*, 6(2), 48–54.

Neill, J. (2002b). Transcendence and transformation in the life patterns of women living with rheumatoid arthritis. *Advances in Nursing Science*, 24(4), 27–47.

Newman, M. A. (1979). *Theory development in nursing*. Philadelphia, PA: F. A. Davis.

Newman, M. A. (1990). Newman's theory of health as praxis. *Nursing Science Quarterly*, 3(1), 37–41.

Newman, M. A. (1994). *Health as expanding consciousness* (2nd ed). New York, NY: National League for Nursing.

Newman, M. A. (1995). Recognizing a pattern of expanding consciousness in persons with cancer. In M. A. Newman, A *developing discipline: Selected works of Margaret Newman* (pp. 159–171). New York, NY: National League for Nursing.

Newman, M. A. (1997). Evolution of the theory of health as expanding consciousness. *Nursing Science Quarterly*, 10(1), 22–25.

Newman, M. A. (1999). Rhythm of relating in a paradigm of wholeness. *Image: The Journal of Nursing Scholarship*, 31(3), 227–229.

Newman, M. A. (2002). Caring in the human health experience. *International Journal for Human Caring*, 6(2), 8–12.

Newman, M. A., Lambe, G. S., & Michaels, C. (1991). Nurse case management: The coming together of theory and practice. *Nursing and Health Care*, 12(8), 404–408.

Noveletsky-Rosenthal, H. T. (1996). Pattern recognition in older adults living with chronic illness. Unpublished doctoral dissertation, Boston College.

Noveletsky-Rosenthal, H., & Solomon, K. (2001). Reflections of the use of John's model of structured reflection in nurse practitioner education. *International Journal for Human Caring*, 4(2), 21–26.

Pharris, M. D. (2002). Coming to know ourselves as community through a nursing partnership with adolescents convicted of murder. *Advances in Nursing Science*, 24(3), 21–42.

Picard, C. (1998). Uncovering pattern of expanding consciousness in midlife women: Creative movement and the narrative as modes of expression. *Dissertation Abstracts International*, 59/03 (UMI No. 9828038).

Picard, C. (2000). Pattern of expanding consciousness in midlife women: Creative movement and the narrative as modes of expression. *Nursing Science Quarterly*, 13(2), 150–158.

Picard, C. (2002). Family reflections of living through sudden death of a child. *Nursing Science Quarterly*, 15(3), 242–250.

Picard, C., Agretelis, J., & DeMarco, R. (2004). Nurse experiences as cancer survivors: Part II–Professional. *Oncology Nursing Forum*, 31(3), 537–542.

Picard, C., & Mariolis, T. (2002). Praxis as a mirroring process: Teaching psychiatric nursing grounded in Newman's health as expanding consciousness. *Nursing Science Quarterly*, 15(2), 118–122.

Schlotzhauer, M., & Farnham, R. (1997). Newman's theory and insulin dependent diabetes mellitus in adolescence. *Journal of School Nursing*, 13(3), 20–23.

Smith, S. K. (1997a). Women's experiences of victimizing sexualization, Part I: Responses related to abuse in home and family environment. *Issues in Mental Health Nursing*, 18, 395–416.

Smith, S. K. (1997b). Women's experiences of victimizing sexualization, Part II: Community and longer term personal impacts. *Issues in Mental Health Nursing*, 18, 417–432.

Tommet, P. A. (2003). Nurse–parent dialogue: Illuminating the evolving pattern of families with children who are medically fragile. *Nursing Science Quarterly*, 16(3), 239–246.

Weingourt, R. (1998). Using Margaret A. Newman's theory of health with elderly nursing home residents. *Perspectives in Psychiatric Care*, 34(3), 25–30.

Yamashita, M. (1999). Newman's theory of health applied in family caregiving in Canada. *Nursing Science Quarterly*, 12(1), 73–79.

Young, A. M. (1976). *The reflexive universe: Evolution of consciousness*. San Francisco, CA: Robert Briggs.

CHAPTER THREE

LINKING NEWMAN'S THEORY OF HEALTH AS EXPANDING CONSCIOUSNESS TO ETHICS AND CARING

CAROLYN HAYES

"I believe that caring is a moral imperative for nursing. Going through the motions of job responsibilities without caring is not nursing." (Newman, 1994, p. 141)

Introduction

In every patient care situation, nurses are accountable for assessing the potential benefits and potential harms of an intervention. To be ethical, the goals of care for an individual patient and his or her family must be determined based on their potential to provide more good than the potential for, or actual, harm. Very few absolutes exist in health care. Therefore, every situation is unique and must be decided contextually. Ethical principles, similar cases, professional codes, position statements, policies, and procedures can all serve as guides, but each case nevertheless remains a collaborative effort to establish the most ethical course of action for that individual client. Most significantly for nurses, our ontologies of person, health, nurse, and environment help guide those decisions. Consequently, as nurses enter into these debates, they need to be clear about the nature of person. This chapter examines the links between ethics, caring, and Newman's theory of health as expanding consciousness (HEC).

The Nature of Person and the Ethic of Care

The American Nurses Association's (ANA) *Social Policy Statement* (2003) presents nursing's view of person when it states, "Humans manifest an essential unity of mind/body/spirit" (p. 3). Unfortunately, there is a tendency to examine the patient situation and healthcare provider options from a prioritization of the individual perspectives of first the person's mind, then his or her body, and then his or her spirit. The emphasis compromises the unity of these aspects of person. The priorities and choices are different when understanding of person and goals of care are viewed from another perspective. Newman offers this view of the person:

> When we begin to think of ourselves as centers of consciousness (patterns of energy) within an overall pattern of expanding conscious- ness, we can begin to see that what we sense of our lives is part of a much larger whole. First the pattern of consciousness that is the person; then broadening the focus, the pattern of consciousness that is the family and physical surroundings; then the pattern that is the communi- ty, the person's larger environmental affiliations, such as work or school; and ultimately the pattern of the world. It is this pattern of the whole that is the phenomenon of Nursing's practice. (Newman, 1994, p. 24)

Imagine a discussion about treatment options, such as surgery versus medica- tion, in which the person is viewed within larger patterns. From Newman's per- spective, "the focus of nursing is on the pattern of the whole, with caring as a moral imperative. As we concentrate on this discipline, our practice and the lives of those we serve will be transformed" (1994, p. xix). Belief in this perspective can lead providers to different therapy decisions and invite/support the client to self- determine using the concept of self. When nurses practice by focusing on the person and honoring the partnership between the nurse and patient, they become conscious of the pattern of the whole and stay focused on meaning.

Newman notes that the "frontal attack on disease failed to bring about sig- nificant changes in our sense of health" (1994, p. 10). Focusing exclusively on technical options and prognostic statistics rather than on person and meaning can also compromise ethical decisions made at the bedside or in the home. The wholeness of the human experience as an essential component of decision making must be recognized, and it must inform decisions and choices as much as the physiological data, whether known or hypothetical.

Framing the Clinical Dialogue: Ethical Approaches

Biomedical ethics emerged to address the question, "What ought we do?" when technology in health care had advanced past our collective moral rea- soning on certain issues. Approaches employed today include principlism, narrative ethics, and care ethics. Unfortunately, most writings and research in ethics to date have targeted on the physician–patient relationship. Nursing's discipline-specific view of person, health, environment, and goals of care are not well represented in these works and subsequent debates.

Gilligan (1982) suggested that ethics should be contextually defined and argued that justice-based reasoning without examination of context and relationships was insufficient. The beginning of care-based reasoning eventually helped healthcare ethics move away from a purely principle-based approach. (See Table 3.1 for definitions of the major principles in biomedical ethics.)

Context and relationships are two core elements commonly examined in clinical ethics today. How else could one begin to explain that for two patients in the exact same physiological state, aggressive therapies are recommended to treat the illness in patient A, while withdrawal of care is selected for patient B? Ideally, it is recognition of each person's uniqueness, wholeness, and pattern within the context of the lived experience that contributes to different treatment options and care outcomes.

Benjamin and Curtis (1992) describe integrity-preserving compromise, a strategy for resolution of ethical conflicts in clinical practice, as occurring in situations of factual uncertainty and moral complexity. It is the very nature of

Table 3.1.	ETHICAL PRINCIPLES
Autonomy	The ethical principle that obliges one to allow individuals to self-determine their own plans and actions. It entails respecting the personal liberty of individuals and the choices they make, based on their own personal values and beliefs.
Beneficence	The ethical principle that obliges one to provide good (e.g., promote someone's welfare) and avoid harm, also known as nonmaleficence (e.g., prevent putting someone at risk for harm).
Justice	The ethical principle that obliges one to treat those who are equal, in relevant respects, in the same manner. When individuals are unequal, in relevant respects, one is obliged to treat them in a fair manner. This means that those who have a greater need may justly receive more of a particular resource than those with a lesser need.
Fidelity	The ethical principle that obliges one to remain faithful to one's commitments, especially the keeping of promises and the protection of confidentiality.
Veracity	The ethical principle that obliges one to tell the truth and to not lie or deceive others.
Confidentiality	The ethical obligation to keep someone's personal and private information secret or private.

pattern—not knowing what is coming next—that creates the sense of uncertainty. Bishop and Scudder (2001) believe that healthcare professionals have turned to ethicists and principles to solve moral problems. These authors argue that nursing is a caring practice and call for a "nursing ethics that takes seriously the meaning inherent in nursing practice" (p. 1). They suggest the development of nursing ethics that is focused on the fulfillment of nursing's moral sense, not merely the application of philosophical ethics to moral problems. Furthermore, these authors challenge all nurses to take seriously the moral intent of nursing practice.

HEC and Ethics

Health as expanding consciousness calls for examination of context and relationships. Newman (1994) used Bateson's conceptualization that a ratio between two quantities is already the beginning of a pattern as a means to explain pattern. In specific cases, clinical ethics is often a process of examining the ratio of harms and benefits. Decisions in health care are often made without full knowledge of what may occur next. Bateson (1979) sees pattern change occurring with new information. Pattern cannot always be predicted with certainty, however, because additional information needed to determine the outcome has not yet happened. Therefore, to make a decision based on what information is known at the moment presents problems in making a choice that is ethical. It is the ratio of harm and benefits as well as an understanding of the person's pattern that will yield the most ethical response. Understanding the nature of person is the key to this reasoning. Not being able to predict pattern is the very source of ethical concern in some clinical situations. That uncertainty exists in the entire system—not just for the one person with whom and for whom, decisions are being made.

HEC as a theory seeks to honor the moral intentions embedded in nursing's social commitment to society. Nursing ethics is not separate from nursing theory anymore than nursing research is separate from HEC-based nursing practice. In addition, the nurse is not separated from the client, nor is the client separated into parts. Wholeness incorporates nursing ethics as a part of the whole of nursing practice. The relationship between the nurse and the patient is the essence of our disciplinary perspective as researchers, theorists, and clinicians.

Newman has described health as more than a dichotomy between health and illness: "We have become idolatrous of health" (1994, p. 4). To place these concepts in opposition limits the meaning of illness within the context of the whole. Newman views illness as an expression of the whole and as a manifestation of health. In the current healthcare environment, we have also become idolatrous of autonomy. Originally, autonomy gained favor when expressed as the patient's right to refuse unwanted treatment. It has grown to be perceived as the absolute guiding ethical principle, nearly voiding the originally strongest held value of nonmaleficence, or doing no harm. In addition, the power of autonomy is now often misconstrued as carrying sufficient moral weight to override the healthcare professional's moral agency. In accepting this view, we have compromised individuals' rights and choices. Just as health and illness cannot be viewed at opposite ends of a continuum, so too ethical principles cannot easily be dichotomized. Ethical principles are interrelated and cannot operate in isolation from the other principles. How can one engage in a beneficent act without including justice? Can one be beneficent and not just? Can I respect someone's autonomy, respect him or her as a person, and yet not explain why I consider something to be beneficent even if he or she does not want it done? Which action demonstrates authentic respect for the person—doing the beneficent act or not doing it because of autonomy concerns? These principles are no more discrete than a person's thoughts, feelings, beliefs, and physical being. We are whole and without acceptance of that wholeness in all we experience, no principle will fully answer all ethical questions.

Applying a dialectical approach may support Hegel's dialectical fusion of opposites, and thinking in terms of a synthesized view may help to see how nurses are making actual ethical decisions. A fusion of all principles is necessary to answer the basic ethical question, "What ought we do?" This question is far more in need of fusion than the technical question, "What can we do?" Just as HEC describes disease as a part of health, so too does beneficence include autonomy. It cannot be beneficial if it is undesired, and vice versa. Autonomy includes beneficence, because action cannot be respectful of another if it is not beneficial. The real question is, "How does this person, as a whole, experience harms and benefits?" This query offers the opportunity for the uniqueness of a person's pattern to become the central focus of the ethical debate. The pattern of the whole is the approach used in nursing ethics to reason and help resolve those dilemmas we confront in clinical situations.

Nursing's Relational Covenant, Care, and Ethics

Fry defines moral accountability as follows:

> . . . being answerable to someone for something one has done or for the responsibilities associated with a particular role assumed by the individual. It includes providing an explanation or rationale according to public standards/norms. . . . The standards/norms of moral accountability are specified by codes of ethics and practice standards (1994, p. 287).

So how does nursing define its role? What covenants have we as nurses created with society?

From its inception, nursing as a distinct discipline has been concerned with holism and the relationship between patient and nurse. Nightingale defined nursing as having "charge of the personal health of somebody . . . and what nursing has to do . . . is to put the patient in the best condition for nature to act upon him" (1859/1992, p. 75). In addition to physical care, Nightingale detailed environmental concerns requiring the nurse's attention, observations that cued the nurse to talk to a patient about the patient versus discussing something else, and examples of existential crises that patients experienced along with the appropriate nurse responses. Nightingale also addressed the mind/ body connection when she said:

> Volumes are now written and spoken upon the effect of the mind upon the body. Much of it is true. But I wish a little more was thought of the effect of the body on the mind. You who believe yourselves overwhelmed with anxieties, but are able every day to walk up Regent Street, or out in the country, to take your meals with others in other rooms, &c., &c., you little know how much your anxieties are thereby lightened; you little know how intensified they become to those who can have no change; how the very walls of their sick rooms seem hung with their care; how the ghosts of their troubles haunt their beds; how impossible it is for them to escape from a pursuing thought without some help from variety. (1859/1992, p. D1)

These early writings highlight the dimensions of care that nurses have always been encouraged to consider—namely, patients' needs beyond the physical realm and within a holistic framework. Reaffirming nursing's commitment to holism, the ANA's *Social Policy Statement* (2003) identified six essential features of professional nursing practice:

- Provision of a caring relationship that facilitates health and healing
- Attention to the full range of experiences and responses to health and illness within the physical and social environment
- Integration of objective data with knowledge gained from an appreciation of the patient's or group's subjective experience
- Application of scientific knowledge to the processes of diagnosis and treatment through the use of judgment and critical thinking
- Advancement of professional nursing knowledge through scholarly inquiry
- Influence on social and public policy to promote social justice (p. 5)

This document extends the roots of holism in nursing practice articulated by Nightingale by stating nursing values and assumes that "Humans manifest as essential unity of mind, body and spirit" (p. 3). Additionally, it advises nurses to consider patients in context while paying attention to changes in roles and relationships.

Bishop and Scudder describe modern nursing practice as holistic care and describe its inherent interactive nature: "Holistic care begins with the patient's first-person experience of illness and nursing care and the nurse's first-person experience of the practice of caring" (2001, p. 35). Again, this statement highlights the dynamic nature of the nurse–patient interaction. The practice of nursing is inherently interactive, and the nurse is intended to receive a benefit—namely, the experience of caring—from the interaction.

The American Association of Critical Care Nurses (AACN) Certification Corporation (1995) also set out to describe nursing practice. The resulting description of nursing at the close of the twenty-first century reflected a practice developed through synergistic relationships with patients. More than 100 years after Nightingale's writings, nursing continues to be described as an interactive, dynamic practice where nurse and patient learn from and experience the other. Nursing is not a prescribed practice—it is interactive and dynamic. Today, nursing is conceptualized as a holistic practice in keeping with the concept of holism advanced by Nightingale and the nurse theorists that followed.

ANA Code for Nurses

The ANA *Code for Nurses with Interpretive Statements* states that "the nurse, in all professional relationships, practices with compassion and respect for the inherent dignity, worth, and uniqueness of every individual, unrestricted by considerations of social or economic status, personal attributes, or the nature of health problems" (2001, p. 4). The statement offers nurses a clear call not only to care *for* recipients of nursing care but also to care *about* them. To further explicate nursing as a relational covenant, the ANA's *Social Policy Statement* states:

> The relationship between a nurse and patient involves participation of both in the process of care. The interaction occurs within the context of the values and beliefs of the patient and the nurse. . . . The values and assumptions apply whether the recipient of professional nursing is an individual, family, group, community or population. (2003, p. 3)

The nurse's values and beliefs are equal in the relationship. It is not a unilateral but rather a mutual process. This mutuality is also described by Newman:

> Nursing intervention is derived from a relational paradigm that directs the professional to enter into a partnership with the client, often at a time of chaos, with the mutual goal of participating in an authentic relationship, trusting that in the process of its unfolding, both will emerge at a higher level of consciousness. (1994, p. 97)

The ANA's 1997 position statement on cultural diversity addressed cultural and spiritual considerations within nursing practice. This document advocates that nurses "understand that nurse–patient encounters include the interaction of three cultural systems: the culture of the nurse, the culture of the client and the culture of the setting" (1997, p. 1). Within this context, the cultures of the nurse and the patient become an important aspect of the care. Nursing covenants call for nurses to provide care that is morally accountable and dependent upon an understanding of context, wholeness, and integration of the nurse as person within descriptions of the relationship with patients.

Resolving Ethical Issues

There is a call for collaboration within nursing's codes and contracts. The eighth statement in the ANA's *Code for Nurses* states, "The nurse collaborates with other health professionals and the public in promoting community, national, and international efforts to meet health needs" (2001, p. 4). Collaborative, interdisciplinary dialogue is needed to answer ethical questions. Clinical ethics requires an examination of the patient's situation through different lenses to capture what is still less than whole, but optimized. We make this examination while incorporating patient, family, and interdisciplinary input. As Newman writes, "We need to remind ourselves that our manifest reality is a small portion of the total enfoldment of the pattern in time-space" (1994, p. 74).

According to Newman (1994), pattern recognition is a mutual process, whereby the nurse reflects his or her own pattern, and after engaging in dialogue with patients and families, comes to together with them to understand and reflect back their pattern of meaning. Given that our codes and position statements mandate relational ethics, in which the nurse's values and beliefs become part of the equation, an understanding of self is necessary. This is a significant part of the nursing context of ethical decision making.

Ethics within HEC Praxis

What are the implications for ethics on practice, research, education, and administration within the HEC theory? There is an assumption that making healthcare decisions helps individuals reach higher levels of consciousness as they seek to understand personal health. Nursing practice recognizes that achieving this recognition requires that the individual become aware of the choices made within the pattern of whole. Guiding the person to a new personal awareness through reflection and dialogue helps him or her to find meaning, interpret experiences, and achieve growth. Personal transformation brought about through insight and self-knowing expands consciousness, as manifested in new behaviors and practices—especially those related to health and lifestyle.

Many examples can be cited in which HEC explains ethical reasoning for nurses. For instance, nursing can use wholeness to frame the seemingly paternalistic approach to pediatric ethics as distinct from ethical decision making for adult patients. As Newman states:

> Pattern manifested by a disease does not stop with one person but is part of the greater whole. In the process of considering the pattern of interaction of an individual with the environment, one inevitably considers the pattern of interaction of the family and the community. (1994, p. 25)

As a society, we protect children from the decisions of others. We may choose not to grant full parental rights if we believe the child may be at risk for harm. As a society, we believe that what happens to one—the child—affects us all. That is the moral premise for state interference. We hold the child's rights in trust as a moral community.

The idea of benevolent deception, withholding truth to avoid harm, such as not telling a patient that he or she is dying, is always difficult to justify. Pattern recognition may help frame potentially conflicting quality-of-life decisions or decisions to withhold information. However, recognizing the best solution to an ethical question posed by a situation may rely less on the thinking of an interdisciplinary team's decision making and more on engaging in a dialogue with the patient that promotes new awareness and fosters greater choice. This approach can honor the right of person to choose and alleviate tensions and conflict.

Nursing is responsible for recognizing the potential that a health or illness situation may present for personal growth and new opportunity. "Recognition of pattern of the whole was pinpointed as the responsibility of nursing science and practice" (Newman, 1994, p. xvi). Through pattern recognition, the nurse intentionally creates an environment of care that optimizes the potential of a situation for choice and expanded consciousness.

Not being able to predict pattern is often the source of moral distress. According to Jameton (1984), moral distress is not being able to do what you know is the right action. Many nurses express frustration because they are often confronted by situations they feel they cannot change. However, moral distress may be reduced when one has a way to gain deeper understanding of wholeness and meaning of personal responses to a situation.

Chambliss (1997) reported that nurses experienced moral distress related to their unique care perspective with patients. He detailed examples of how differently nurses saw patient situations. For example, nurses were expected to initiate cardiopulmonary resuscitation even though they did not believe it was the right thing to do. They did not have one of the two "power buttons," the autonomy held by the patient/family or the authority held by the physician to determine medical futility during the decision-making process. Not empowered to decide, the nurse becomes the agent of an act he or she finds morally wrong, and must begin resuscitation efforts and call for the rest of the team.

When nurses understand their unique vantage point on the moral distress present in a situation, it may guide their decisions related to the resuscitation efforts or assuage their conviction that it is the wrong action to take. As Newman suggests:

> Viewed from the perspective of the larger pattern, the activity of partic-ular foci are understood in terms of the activity of the total system. Clusters of alliances change in relation to the tasks that need to be done. When one comprehends the whole, knowledge of the parts becomes meaningful. . . . The paradox is that the whole can be seen in the parts. A specific event can be viewed as an example of a class of events, and in this way the most specific patterns of a person may serve as prototypes of the general overall pattern of the person. There is generality in the specific. (1994, p. 75)

The ANA's *Social Policy Statement* (2003) can be interpreted using the framework of HEC to yield new insights. For example, the definitions of health and illness as human experiences can be seen as being commensurate with the idea that health and disease are not dichotomized concepts: "The presence of illness does not preclude health, nor does optimal health preclude illness" (p. 3).

Newman's attention to wholeness also refers to Bohm's (1980) concept of holomovement, the unitary and continuous nature of person within the undi-vided whole of the universe through time and space. This idea offers another explanation for much of clinical ethics. It explains why clinicians concern them-selves with professional ethics, and it acknowledges the awareness that deci-sions made in a particular case reflect the values of the larger professional community because of potential erosions of public trust. When clinicians par-ticipate in decision making within the context of a larger whole, they recognize the present while also considering the impact of the past and on the future. That thinking provides an example of how nurses can transcend time and space as they provide care.

Holomovement also explains patient decision making. It provides an op-portunity to question how present decisions are informed by past choices and, in turn, influence future actions. As Newman stated:

> Nowhere is the conflict of different time patterns more evident than in the bureaucratic system of the hospital. The timing of activities within a complex system such as a large hospital is indeed an intricate task and has become even more intense with the shortened hospital stays imposed by the cost-cutting strategies. (1994, p. 53)

This issue remains valid, in both acute care and home care. Nursing practice guided by HEC assumes the cultivation of nursing presence to the one being cared for in partnership. In Chapter 1, Newman defined the nature of nursing practice as being fully in the present to embrace the meaning of the situation for the person. It is a challenge for some nurses to move toward *being with* as comfortably as they move toward *action*.

How can we use HEC to guide nursing time spent with the patient so as to add or enhance the intention of expanding consciousness? The exploration of the meaning of time, the provision of opportunities for dialogue and sharing of meaning, and the experience of both the nurse and the patient may be conceptualized as just. It may be the most morally accountable thing our discipline could attend to at this point in time. The ability of the nurse to know the patient and be aware of the stressors that hospitalization brings to the person can result in changing the environment of care to one that embraces both the uniqueness and the wholeness of the person and one that optimizes rather than compromises healing.

Questions of informed consent also take on new dimensions when viewed from within the HEC theoretical model. Patterns associated with decision making, information processing and capacity for integration all influence an individual's choice to seek help and take action. A person's usual fear responses, pattern of control, and sense of self can underlie a decision to act. Understanding the person's usual responses to stressful and potentially threatening situations can help frame the way a nurse approaches the individual to discuss informed consent. For example, a person who pattern of decision- making relies heavily on having all of the facts before proceeding with an action may require extensive teaching and clarification before agreeing to an intervention.

It is therefore unethical to approach all patients the same way for informed consent. When considering informed consent, HEC would direct us to understand that limitations in movement, impact a person's sense of time and timing. If the clinician is sensitive to the person's pattern, they will work to be in synchrony with that pattern as they share information. This enhances the patient's capacity to process the information and make their decisions regarding consent.

Exemplar

Setting: An ethics rounds at a major teaching hospital. As I sat there, listening intently, participating passionately, I couldn't help but notice, my worldview is radically different. Others spoke of autonomy, beneficence, non-maleficence and societal obligations of healthcare providers as mechanistically as I make out a grocery list. We were talking about actively ending lives. I heard references to the patient not really 'being there anymore anyway'. What does that mean? When does a patient stop being a person?

The Debate

The theoretical debate was about euthanasia. The debate was about something with which we all had been confronted in our practice. Upon reflection, I recognized that moment as transformative. My perspective is not without solid foundation in law and in nursing ethics. I could easily argue against it from traditional principles or the law. The Supreme Court ruling in 1997 affirmed a distinction between intentionally hastening death and use of means to alleviate pain even if it hastens death. The principle of "double effect" is supported in ANA position statements to which I could defer, but those arguments skim the surface of a more deeply held belief: a respect for persons that allows for the person to be different than he or she was before, inclusive of disease, still person, still whole.

Linking Debate to HEC

My ethical perspective is informed by HEC. In a lecture I presented on nursing ethics at end of life, I concluded with a quote from Margaret Newman that articulates that belief:

> To be open is to be vulnerable, an important characteristic of human-ness. To be vulnerable is often to suffer. We tend to avoid suffering, and yet avoidance of suffering may deter movement to higher levels of consciousness. Suffering offers us the opportunity to transcend a particular situation. Vulnerability, suffering, disease, death do not diminish us. What does diminish us is trying to protect ourselves by binding ourselves off from those experiences. The need is to let go, embrace our experience, and allow the expansion of consciousness to unfold. (1994, p. 142)

My passionate belief in that statement, rather than the principles of ethics, frames my opinions about euthanasia. People must be given the opportunity to let their consciousness expand. Hastening death, sparing loved ones from witnessing suffering, and other such measures run counter to that belief. We interrupt the opportunity to transcend the situation. We do not recognize wholeness in the disease. We do not accept that the person is energy in constant exchange with the environment despite his or her inability to cognitively respond to us. The arguments I heard in the room during my lecture could be rephrased to say, "We cannot *do* anything else, so clearly this patient is no longer a person." Is it our hubris, our need *to do*, which creates the tension that is strong enough to stop seeing another as a person?

What if this altered state, unreachable by our traditional means, is actually the highest level of consciousness? There exists a possible paradox that un-consciousness may be the highest level of consciousness attainable while still in physical form. Bentov's (1978) analogy of ice and steam as alternate forms of water is one way to examine our preconceptions of unconscious patients. We cannot identify with certainty the moment when "movement and rest fuse into one" (p. 67). Given the constant energy exchange, would we not want to be present with this person as long as possible? Selfishly perhaps, we see the potential to gain from the exchange. We allow the person an opportunity to leave a lasting legacy. Conversely, if this is a lower level of consciousness, then by remaining with the patient we continue to serve in the exchange. An ethical worldview, informed by Newman's theory of expanding consciousness, is a solid foundation on which to base a caring and ethical nursing practice.

References

AACN Certification Corporation (1995). Redefining nursing according to patients' and families' needs: An evolving concept. AACN *Clinical Issues*, 6(1), 153–156.

American Nurses Association (1997). *Position statement on cultural diversity in nursing practice*. Washington, DC: American Nurses Publishing.

American Nurses Association (2001). *Code for nurses with interpretive statements*. Washington, DC: American Nurses Publishing.

American Nurses Association (2003). *Social policy statement* (2nd ed.). Washington, DC: American Nurses Publishing.

Bateson, G. (1979). *Mind and nature: A necessary unity*. Toronto: Bantam.

Benjamin, M., & Curtis, J. (1992). *Ethics in nursing* (3rd ed.). New York, NY: Oxford University Press.

Bentov, I. (1978). *Stalking the wild pendulum*. New York: E. P. Dutton.

Bishop, A. H., & Scudder, J. R. (2001). *Nursing ethics: Holistic caring practice*. Sudbury, MA: Jones and Bartlett.

Bohm, D. (1980). *Wholeness and the implicate order*. London: Routledge & Kegan Paul.

Chambliss, D. (1997). *Beyond caring: Hospitals, nurses, and the social organization of ethics*. Chicago, IL: University of Chicago Press.

Fry, S. (1994). *Ethics in nursing practice*. Geneva, Switzerland: International Council of Nurses.

Gilligan, C. (1982). *In a different voice: Psychological theory and women's development*. Cambridge, MA: Harvard University Press.

Jameton, A. (1984). *Nursing practice, the ethical issues*. Englewood, NJ: Prentice-Hall.

Newman, M. A. (1994). *Health as expanding consciousness* (2nd ed.). New York, NY: National League for Nursing.

Nightingale, F. (1859/1992). *Notes on nursing*. Philadelphia, PA: J. B. Lippincott.

PART TWO
CARING PRAXIS

Suffering, Growth, and Possibility: Health as Expanding Consciousness in End-of-Life Care

Anne-Marie Barron

Introduction

Application of Newman's theory of health as expanding consciousness (HEC) in research and clinical practice can optimize end-of-life care. In *Life Meanings and the Experience of Cancer* (Barron, 2001) the author uses Newman's theoretical orientation and research protocol to help explain this experience from the perspective of the clinician and the patient. This chapter discusses connections made during the study with participants and staff and also reflect on Newman's influence on my current clinical practice.

A Professional Narrative

During my early clinical experience as a psychiatric liaison nurse, opportunities frequently arose to work with patients who had cancer, their families, and the staff who cared for them. Many of these patients described a quest for meaning and purpose in the cancer experience. Working with them, I came to understand that critical attributes of spirituality included an intentional examination of ultimate values, personal knowing, and inner strength (Barron, 1997). These patients seemed to put their suffering into a larger perspective to make it more bearable. Surprisingly, some of them talked about the "gift" of cancer in their lives. Patients made profound changes in their relationships and work lives as a result of developing a deeper sense of meaning and life. They often experienced great personal growth during this period.

In my role as a liaison nurse, I facilitated support groups for cancer patients. Group participants considered the meaning of their illnesses, lives, and possible deaths. They recognized the importance of establishing and sustaining relationships based on love, acceptance, and forgiveness. Relationships with important others—spouses, children, and parents—often grew and flourished because of this enhanced appreciation of person. Group members made important changes in their work, based on new understandings of purpose and meaning. For example, one young man with metastatic melanoma decided to leave his work as a farmer and become a minister. He completed seminary and was serving as a minister in a church at the time of his death, many years after receiving a bleak prognosis. Another support-group member, a young woman with acute leukemia, decided to leave teaching and become a social worker. She became the director of a hospice and then established a private practice. Despite having a very poor prognosis for five-year survival, she is now, more than 25 years later, considered cured.

The commitment, strength, and caring that guided the connections within the group were profound. Members of this support group helped one another to live more fully and sometimes to die, becoming ever more whole, more fully human, and connected to one another and to what was most important to them.

Along the way, I came to appreciate that end of life was a time of growth and possibility. I often said to colleagues that some of the healthiest people I knew were dying! My living was richer and more intentional for having worked with these patients. I understood more deeply the meaning of love, forgiveness, and purpose. I knew I was experiencing profound aspects of the human experience and the deepest aspects of nursing practice. At the same time, I had no clear theoretical orientation to understand it all. When members of the support group wanted to focus on the spiritual meaning of their illnesses, I was relieved that the door to the meeting room was closed. I wondered what my colleagues would have thought about my practice if they happened to listen in on the conversation. Simultaneously, I recognized that these group discussions helped to shift life perspectives for all involved, and made suffering more bearable.

When I returned to graduate school for doctoral study, I wanted to focus my research in some way on gaining further understanding of spirituality and the cancer experience. I knew that although my patients had very serious disease processes, they continued to flourish as people. As I became acquainted with HEC theory, I recognized that I had been offering caring in the human health experience. I began my journey with a concept analysis of spirituality. The work of many nursing authors (Barnum, 1996; Burkhardt, 1989, 1994; Emblen, 1992; Highfield, 1991; Macrae, 1995; Nagai-Jacobson & Burkhardt, 1989; Reed, 1987, 1991a, 1991b, 1992; Stuart, Deckro & Mandle, 1989; Roberts & Whall, 1996) deepened my understanding of spirituality and helped to clarify my prior clinical experience. The next step was to design a research study that would elucidate understanding of spirituality in the experience of cancer. HEC helped to shape my understanding of the phenomena of my research interest more clearly.

Relevant HEC Concepts

Newman's theory views humans as unitary beings, irreducible, indivisible, multidimensional, and unfolding in an undivided universe (Newman, 1994, 1995a, 1997a, 1997b). Each person has a unique pattern, which includes genetic patterns as well as movement, diversity, rhythm, energy exchange, and transformation. Pattern is expressed in meaningful relatedness to others and the environment. Health is an evolving process of developing self-awareness and insight within the larger context of the environment and with increasing ability to perceive alternatives and varieties of response. "Health is viewed as the evolving pattern of the whole, the explication of the unfolding implicate order" (Newman, 1994, pp. 82–83).

Identifying pattern is the essence of nursing practice. Nurses become therapeutic partners with patients searching for pattern and meaning, with understanding serving as an impetus toward growth and expansion of consciousness. According to Newman, in a therapeutic relationship, the nurse and the patient form a unified whole. She uses the analogy of throwing two stones into the water, where each stone forms an initial interference pattern in the water; as the patterns connect, a larger pattern that contains both patterns forms. In a therapeutic relationship, the nurse often experiences the pattern of the patient and can share insights regarding the person's expression of pattern. It is critical that the nurse recognizes his or her capacity to serve as a mirror for the patient, and understands that the nurse's experience within the relationship reflects the whole. The goal of the interaction is for the patient to recognize and understand the meaning of his or her own pattern. In the therapeutic process, the nurse is fully present and participates in a transformational process as meaning unfolds. Change is unpredictable and may be experienced as disruptive and disorganizing before moving toward organization. Both nurse and patient are changed in the process.

Research Methodology

Newman's perspective on qualitative methodology involves the nurse researcher as an integral part of an interaction pattern that supports the process of pattern recognition and choice. This method has the following elements: establishing mutuality; focusing on the most meaningful events and people in the participant's life; organizing the data and diagramming the data as sequential patterns over time; and sharing the data with the participant for confirmation or revision (Newman, 1994). HEC-grounded dialogue and reflection on pattern provides an opportunity for insight, which can lead to choice and action possibilities. The result: nursing praxis.

As I deepened my understanding of HEC, the purpose of my research became clear—to further understand patterns, meaning perspectives, expanding consciousness, and spirituality in the experience of cancer. A goal was to generate knowledge about the process of praxis as well as understanding participants' stories and meaning that could inform nursing practice and ultimately lead to the alleviation of suffering. Within HEC theory, suffering can be viewed as an impetus for change and transformation. Meaning and understanding can lead to acceleration of evolving consciousness. Suffering might also be considered central to wholeness, health, and expanding consciousness. As persons suffer, turbulence and chaos are created. Yet within turbulence and chaos, growth is possible. Exploring the connections between meaning, pattern, and spirituality seemed to offer the possibility of further understanding of how that transformation occurs.

Three research questions were developed. The first question was consistent with Newman's methodology:

1. How do persons with cancer express meaning over time?

Additional questions, using a phenomenologic perspective were:

2. What facilitates or hinders expansion of consciousness in persons with cancer?
3. How is spirituality manifested in the narratives of persons with cancer?

Twenty-two adults of varying ages, ethnic backgrounds, and religious backgrounds, all diagnosed with cancer and either receiving care in their homes or hospitalized in an acute care or rehabilitation hospital, formed the study sample. Most participants had advanced forms of cancer.

Findings

The process of engaging in the study was very moving. Participants generously offered to become part of the study because they believed it would ultimately benefit others. The love, courage, compassion, and grace they demonstrated and shared were incredible. Many of the participants were very ill, and several were close to death. Their hope was to ease the suffering of others. They openly and generously shared their experiences and lives with me. The meaning and growth they experienced as a result of the challenges and suffering they endured were inspirational. I am changed by the wisdom and love they shared.

The participants described turbulence and chaos as a result of their en-counters with serious illness, but also shared profound insights and deep personal understandings. They appreciated the opportunity offered by the study to engage in deep reflection and pattern recognition. The patterns iden-tified were meaningful, but perhaps even more meaningful was the process of relationship with the participants and staff at the agencies where the dialogues took place. As Newman described, in the early studies using HEC an overall pattern could be identified, "but in retrospect, this aspect was not as important in guiding nursing practice as the process that transpired between the nurse and the participant in the transformative unfolding" (Newman, 2002, p. 9). A number of nurse researchers also emphasized the importance of caring con-nections, specifically, that resulted from using the HEC research framework (Litchfield, 1999; Endo et al., 2000; Pharris, 2002; Neill, 2002).

Exemplar: Carol

Carol was a woman in her sixties. Eight months before we met, she had been di-agnosed with advanced, metastatic cancer. She was very sick when I interviewed her. Her voice was so soft that the tape recorder did not pick up her descriptions clearly. I paraphrased the interview from my notes and what I could glean from the recording. Carol died several days after our first interview, so I could not share my summary of her life and pattern with her. Although she did not complete the research protocol, she was very much a participant and highly engaged in the study. Because of the urgency of her situation, we focused on her current circumstances rather than the course of her entire life. I will present what unfolded in this limited, but meaningful, encounter.

Due to a recent back surgery to relieve spinal cord compression resulting from the metastatic disease, Carol had been hospitalized for rehabilitation. Unfortunately, the surgery was unsuccessful and she remained paralyzed below her waist. The plan was to offer rehabilitation and then discharge her to her daughter's home. She was very close to this daughter and her son, both of whom were major sources of support.

Carol opened the interview by saying that she had been waiting for someone to ask what was important to her. She explained that she had stopped eating and drinking that morning because she felt that death was near and she did not want to die a long and agonizing death. She thought that withholding nourishment and fluid would hasten the dying process. She was not afraid of death, she explained, but the process of dying terrified her.

Although not in physical pain, Carol was clearly suffering with intense anxiety. In fact, fear of uncontrollable anxiety during the dying process was one of her greatest concerns. The past few years had been filled with emo-tional pain for her. Four years earlier, she had found her husband several hours after he died from a self-inflicted gunshot wound to the head. The couple had just come through a difficult marital period, and she thought they had resolved some troubling issues. His death was shocking and painful to her for many reasons. She did not know what his death had been like or how long he suffered after shooting himself. Although professionals and friends had reassured her that he could not have survived long with the injuries he sustained, the memory of his death haunted her and was heightened as she faced her own death.

Carol had just been getting back on track emotionally when she was diagnosed with advanced cancer. The last few months had been grueling for her. She had been given a prognosis following the recent surgery of 6 to 12 months, but she felt that the prognosis was incorrect and that death was imminent. She asked very difficult questions: "What will it be like with no further nourishment?" "Where am I in relation to illness and death?" "What can be done for my anxiety?" "What medications am I currently taking?" I could not answer her questions. I asked her if she would like me to share her concerns with her nurses and doctors so that they could begin to address her unresolved issues. She very much wanted me to talk with them.

I spoke with the nurse manager and physicians' assistant on the unit about Carol's concerns. The physicians' assistant said that recent data he was compiling suggested that her assessment was accurate and that death was near. As we were discussing Carol's situation, her daughter called the unit. The physicians' assistant shared her mother's concerns and arranged a family meeting for that afternoon. The nurse manager compassionately talked with Carol about her death and her fears. She explained that a comfortable death was the staff's top priority and that they would remain with her throughout the process. They would move her to a private room so that her family could stay with her. She assured Carol of the availability of medications for pain and anxiety and emphasized the staff's commitment to finding the right medications to keep her comfortable.

As a result, Carol became visibly calmer. She asked me to sit with her for a little while, while she slept. After about 30 minutes, she told me that she was feeling much calmer and was ready for me to leave. We set up an appointment for a second research interview. She thanked me for focusing on what was important with her.

The nurse manager called me the morning I was supposed to return and explained that Carol had died the day before. Peacefully praying, she slipped into death as her minister sang her favorite hymn. The minister expressed surprise regarding the unusually peaceful and quiet way that she had died. The minister said she had never been with someone who passed so peacefully into death. Given the intensity of Carol's suffering during our first interview, I had not had the opportunity to reflect on the whole of her life with her. I had tentatively identified a pattern, but since she cannot validate it, my conclusion remains tentative. The pattern identified was direct and strong; gracious and caring; taking charge and maintaining control. Her husband's suicide seemed to disconnect her from that pattern and contributed to the anguish she described during our first encounter. Focusing on what was most important to her allowed her to directly ask for help. Once her anguish and terror were identified and addressed, she could re-engage the directness, grace, and strength that were perhaps reflective of her overall pattern through life.

Exemplar of Researcher–Staff Connection

The second exemplar relates to the relationship of the researcher to unit staff during this data collection period. One day during the study, I casually asked one of the oncology unit nurses, "How are you doing?" This experienced nurse replied, "Not very well, actually." We talked for a bit. She told me about a recent emergency she had experienced. A young patient on the unit had begun to bleed severely, and the nurse immediately recognized that the patient's tumor had eaten through a major artery. She began applying pressure and called for help. Soon the nurse was actually in the bed applying pressure. The bleeding was so intense that she needed to kneel directly over the patient to gain leverage to apply enough pressure to make a difference. Emergency surgery was arranged—but in the midst of a very busy surgical day, it took some time to ready the surgical staff and prepare an operating room. The nurse had to continue to apply intense pressure. She and the patient were actually wheeled together in his bed from the unit to the operating room. His life was saved, perhaps for a few precious weeks or months. The nurse knew it was an important time for him. She was very pleased that he would have more time to say good-bye. When she closed her eyes, however, she saw the terror in his eyes and relived the agonizing attempt to slow the bleeding. Her heart was filled. The pain of the situation had stayed with her. This nurse was not eating and, when she did sleep, she dreamed about this encounter with profound suffering. We talked, and our dialogue helped the nurse to process her personal distress related to giving care.

The following week I learned that my youngest study participant's bone marrow transplant was not likely to be successful. He was a young man filled with the hopes and dreams of a 22-year-old. His enthusiastic, wise-beyond-his-years reflections and keen sense of both the important and the absurd reminded me of my own son. My heart ached for him, and for his mother. I was filled with sadness. I found that nurse whom I had helped earlier and we talked. Our dialogue helped me to feel comforted in my sadness in the role as researcher.

These connections with the study participant and the nurse were rich encounters. I knew them only in relation to collecting data for my study. The deeply caring nature of the research process seemed to create caring energy that allowed for very meaningful encounters that transcended the specifically focused and time-limited nature of the apparent research relationship.

Informing Clinical Practice and HEC

When returning to clinical practice, my goal was to continue to share the insights gained through research that helped me understand the human experience of health and suffering. I met with the chief of oncology in one of my research settings to share my findings. He invited me to join the staff at his institution and noted the value of my research to practice. I became a part-time clinical nurse specialist and now work regularly with the nurses with whom I had connected so meaningfully during the study. My position was designed to support the retention of new nursing staff on the unit. About the time I started the position, 10 new graduates were hired. Until the nursing shortage arose several years ago, new graduates were not hired there because the practice is so complex and demanding. The shortage necessitated a change, but the nursing leadership recognized that the challenges faced by new graduates in caring for patients with cancer had proved overwhelming for a number of the new nurses. I would help to support them in their roles as new clinicians. My goals in this position are to contribute to the psychosocial dimension of nursing practice and to enhance nursing staff understanding of the research process. Ideally, the position will contribute to the ongoing development of expert nursing practice and foster professional satisfaction on the unit. My initial emphasis has been on clinical practice.

I have been on the unit eight hours per week for almost two years. It has been a rich and meaningful experience for me. I meet regularly with new graduate nurses, consult with the nurses on many complex patient situations, and have begun regular reflective practice rounds. I discuss patients and issues in care with the nurses, and work directly with patients and families and assist with challenging assessments and psychosocial nursing interventions. Early on in the position as I was seeing patients and began offering therapeutic touch for patients to promote comfort and healing. The nurses on the unit requested the opportunity to learn this nursing intervention. I conducted workshops, and now 13 nurses are prepared to provide this modality of care, which cultivates being fully present to the patient.

When asked to see patients and families, I introduce myself as a clinical nurse specialist with a focus on understanding what is most important to patients and families as they receive care during complex and challenging experiences. This statement of purpose has been appreciated and fosters therapeutic engagement and trust. While I do not generally reflect on the patient's whole life to understand pattern, I often develop an understanding of pattern in a general way. A deliberate focus on meaning invites deep connectedness and understanding. From this sense of connectedness, unconditional love and acceptance naturally evolve. When the patient and I have an appreciation of pattern and knowing what is important to that individual, it is possible to appreciate the meaning of behaviors that from a more superficial perspective may seem troublesome or difficult. Intentional presence helps to clarify meaning and possibility, and consciousness is expanded. In this relationship of deep connectedness, suffering can be ameliorated.

Excellent nursing care is offered on the unit where I practice. The nurses are very clearly committed to caring. As one of the chaplains on the unit has said, the nurses *hold* patients and families in the most difficult of circumstances. Exquisite care was being offered before I began my work on the unit, and I feel a sense of pride at becoming a member of such a compassionate and expert team. What I hope my practice brings to the unit is an intentional focus on the deepest aspects of our work nurses' relationship with people and additional opportunities to share the wisdom, challenges, and burdens that encounters with suffering and dying demand.

Conclusions

End-of-life care is enhanced by a HEC perspective. It offers a praxis model of engagement for the researcher or clinician. Nurses engage in reflection, whether in individual encounters or on formal rounds, and are connected more deeply. From that deeper knowing, we see one another more clearly, accept one another without conditions, and infuse our relationships with love and care. As staff, we step back and see the flow and turbulence for patients, for families, and for ourselves. We identify crises and decision-making points. We see patterns, meanings, and possibilities and become more whole, more compassionate, and more fully human. We offer deeper caring, become therapeutic partners for our patients, and participate in a mutual process of transformation and expanding consciousness. Newman's theory of HEC offers a way to understand the deepest aspects of human experience and the profound nature of nursing caring.

References

Barnum, B. (1996). *Spirituality in nursing*. New York, NY: Springer.

Barron, A. M. (1997). *Concept analysis of spirituality*. Unpublished manuscript, Boston College.

Barron, A. M. (2001). Life meanings and the experience of cancer. *Dissertation Abstracts International*, 54(01), 3B (UMI No. 30-08589).

Burkhardt, M. (1989). Spirituality: An analysis of the concept. *Holistic Nursing Practice*, 3(3), 69–77.

Burkhardt, M. (1994). Becoming and connecting: Elements of spirituality for women. *Holistic Nursing Practice*, 8(4), 12–21.

Emblen, J. (1992). Religion and spirituality defined according to use in the nursing literature. *Journal of Professional Nursing, 8*(1), 41–47.

Endo, E., Nitta, N., Inayoshi, M., Saito, R., Takemura, K., & Minegishi, H. (2000). Pattern recognition as a caring partnership in families with cancer. *Journal of Advanced Nursing, 32*(3), 603–610.

Highfield, M. (1991). Spiritual health of oncology patients—nurse and patient perspectives. *Cancer Nursing, 15,* 1–8.

Litchfield, M. (1999). Practice wisdom. *Advances in Nursing Science, 22*(2), 62–73.

Macrae, J. (1995). Nightingale's spiritual philosophy. *Image: The Journal of Nursing Scholarship, 27,* 8–10.

Nagai-Jacobson, M., & Burkhardt, M. (1989). Spirituality: Cornerstone of holistic practice. *Holistic Nursing Practice, 3*(3), 18–26.

Neill, J. (2002). Transcendence and transformation in the life patterns of women living with rheumatoid arthritis. *Advances in Nursing Science, 24*(4), 27–47.

Newman, M. A. (1994). *Health as expanding consciousness* (2nd ed.). New York: National League for Nursing.

Newman, M. A. (1995). A *developing discipline*. New York: National League for Nursing.

Newman, M. A. (1997a). Evolution of the theory of health as expanding consciousness. *Nursing Science Quarterly, 10*(3), 22–25.

Newman, M. A. (1997b). Experiencing the whole. *Advances in Nursing Science, 20*(1), 34–39.

Newman, M. A. (2002). Caring in the human health experience. *International Journal of Human Caring, 6,* 8–11.

Pharris, M. D. (2002). Coming to know ourselves as community through a nursing partnership with adolescents convicted of murder. *Advances in Nursing Science, 24*(3), 21–42.

Reed, P. (1987). Spirituality and well-being in terminally ill hospitalized adults. *Research in Nursing and Health, 10,* 335–344.

Reed, P. (1991a). Preferences for spiritually related nursing interventions among terminally ill and non-terminally ill hospitalized adults and well adults. *Applied Nursing Research, 4*(3), 122–128.

Reed, P. (1991b). Toward a theory of self-transcendence: Deductive reformulation using developmental theories. *Advances in Nursing Science, 13*(4), 64–77.

Reed, P. (1992). An emerging paradigm for the investigation of spirituality in nursing. *Research in Nursing and Health, 15,* 349–357.

Roberts, K., & Whall, A. (1996). Serenity and nursing practice. *Image, 28*(4), 359–364.

Stuart, E., Deckro, J., & Mandle, C. (1989). Spirituality in health and healing: A clinical program. *Holistic Nursing Practice, 3*(3), 35–46.

CHAPTER FIVE

CREATING A HEALING ENVIRONMENT FOR STAFF AND PATIENTS IN A PRE-SURGERY CLINIC

JANE FLANAGAN

Introduction

The goal of this chapter is to describe a model of care grounded in Newman's theory of health as expanding consciousness (HEC). The development of this nursing practice model reflects an evolving, multidimensional process that involves several intersecting phases, interconnected and influencing one another. Although this process has no specific initial or concluding facet, several elements have emerged as essential to creation of a healing environment in the pre-surgical unit: research, vision, commitment, leadership, and mentoring. The development and implementation of the healing environment is, in part, linked to changes within the larger healthcare system. Within this context, the nursing leadership's vision has recognized the unique role played by the nurse and the need to illuminate nursing practice within a competitive healthcare arena. In addition, the team in the pre-surgical clinic has recognized a need for linking nursing care and research so as to distinguish the role of the nurse from that of other healthcare providers.

The Preadmission Nursing Practice Model

The Preadmission Nursing Practice Model (PNPM) was designed to create an opportunity for the authentic relationship between the patient and the nurse to evolve. To date, no known models of care in the perioperative setting have purposefully developed a strategy to foster interaction between the patient and the nurse. The PNPM includes four phases: (1) development, (2) implementation, (3) evaluation, and (4) outcome (Flanagan, 2002). The first two phases of development and implementation center on the strategies needed to advance the PNPM and are the focus of this chapter. This process took place over a two-year period. Critical to the development of this model was the careful attention paid to the impact of knowledge development in nursing and, in particular, the influence of Rogerian science and the work of Margaret Newman.

The Environment of Care: Beginnings

Standard preoperative care includes multidisciplinary assessments and teaching by nursing, anesthesia, and surgical residents. Prior to 1990, patients were admitted the day prior to surgery to receive this care. To save costs, however, insurance companies sought to eliminate this pre-procedure day. Nursing administration within the organization (Massachusetts General Hospital, Boston, MA) recognized a continued need to prepare patients for surgery. As a result, the preadmission clinic (PAC) was introduced in 1990, creating a space for nursing, anesthesia, and surgical residents to provide such care.

Originally, the preadmission clinic was established to assess a small group of same-day surgical admissions. This group included a mix of surgical patients (both by procedure and acuity) who had been denied a preoperative overnight stay by their insurance companies. The PAC quickly expanded to include a larger number of patients planning same-day surgical hospital admissions as well as patients having ambulatory surgery. In one year, the number of patients seen in the clinic rose from about 15 to 40 patients per day. Currently, the clinic prepares 50–60 patients each day for surgery. Since its inception, nurses, surgeons, and anesthesiologists identified a need to provide preoperative surgical preparation to all surgical patients—approximately 125 people each day from both ambulatory surgical service and same-day surgery admissions.

Initially, nurses practicing in this environment used a problem-focused orientation to assess the patients during the preadmission visit. With each patient encounter, nurses identified patient responses to the event using nursing diagnosis (Gordon, 1997; North American Nursing Diagnosis Association, 1999). This action was supported by clinical studies describing negative patient experiences during the perioperative experience amenable to nursing care. Patient responses included ineffective pain management, social isolation, fatigue, and self-care needs (Jones, Coakley & Flanagan, 1999; Jones, Dauphinee, Coakley & Fernsebner, 1998). As a result of the study findings and dialogue with the unit leadership, the nurses in this preadmission clinic came to recognize the importance of nursing presence in achieving improved patient care outcomes. What became clear to all involved was that nurses recognize the uniqueness of person and the need for patients to share their stories. This realization led to the discussions about practice and the desire to develop and articulate the unique focus of nursing in the preadmission setting.

The Process of Model Development and Implementation

The PNPM was initiated by a shift in the philosophical and ontological beliefs about person and nursing, health, and environment for nurses practicing in the preadmission clinic. This personal and professional development of the nursing staff led to the generation of the PNDM model. There was no specific order to the process that emerged, as each step was intertwined with the others. The development and implementation of the PNPM was integral and synchronous (see Table 5.1). The nurses identified the stimuli for change as a personal perception of turmoil, dissatisfaction with current practice, a desire for change, an interest in research and theory-based practice, and the availability of mentoring. All were equally important elements and integral to the process of PNPM development.

The Development Phase of Initiation: Behind Closed Doors

Because the preadmission clinic was expanding so quickly, space was of critical importance. Nurses working in the PAC were often forced to interview patients wherever they could find a somewhat private area. A new clinic was built to respond to the growing demand for preoperative preparation and patient growth. In the new setting, each nurse had an office. While this transition may have seemed subtle, it ultimately had a profound impact on nursing practice in the PAC. For the first time, the nurses had a private space to meet with patients. As a result of this seemingly minor alteration, the delivery of care was changed. Nurses reported less distraction and an ability to focus more on the patient than on the surrounding environment. They began to notice that patients wanted to share personal stories that reflected more than just illness or impending surgery. Within a quiet environment of care, nurses were able to establish an intentional relationship with the patient and to notice how this interaction was changing their practice.

The Development Phase of Initiation: Recognizing the Opportunity

Each PAC nurse was given an opportunity to participate in research investigations with a small group of outpatients having minor surgical procedures. While the nurses in the clinic originally felt they had prepared patients well

Table 5.1.   THE DEVELOPMENT AND IMPLEMENTATION PHASES OF THE
PRE-ADMISSION NURSING PRACTICE MODEL

Development	*Initiation: Behind closed doors*—recognizing the uniqueness of the nurse within the patient interaction.
	Initiation: Recognizing the opportunity—an awareness, openness, and willingness to reexamine practice. This is a vulnerable period because once the need for change becomes apparent, it is difficult not to move forward to explore new ideas.
	Transition: Mission of nursing explored—a period in which nurses reflect on the practice and the way it had been and explore new ways it could be.
	Transition: Linking theory to practice—a period in which nurses draw from theories and ideas that could be implemented in practice and are congruent with their own ideas.
	Transition: Creating the environment of care—a period in which nurses enhance the physical space of the work area to make it more inviting to patients.
Implementation	*Changing practice*—a period in which nurses commit to the new practice ideas and actually implement them into their setting.
	Mentoring—a process in which nurses individually or in team meetings review and discuss practice changes.
	Reflection—a required part of the process, that allows nurses to center prior to and after meeting with patients.
	Coming to know the patient—allowing the patient to share his or her story as suggested by Newman's method (1994).

for postoperative recovery at home, research findings previously mentioned gave the nurses some knowledge of the perioperative experience from the patient's perspective. After these findings were shared with the staff, several PAC nurses volunteered to participate in a study and identified patient responses to outpatient surgery at 24 and 72 hours postoperatively.

The results of this study validated that patients valued nurses' presence and the opportunities they were given to be "known" by the nurses. The study also found that patients reported not being prepared for what to expect during recovery at home, despite the fact that nurses in the preadmission clinic gave the patients "adequate" information. Findings also suggested that more could be accomplished during the preadmission nurse–patient interaction. As a result, nurses in the PAC looked for new ways to make changes in their practice. They returned to issues raised previously during small group staff meetings and discussed patients' desire to tell their stories to the nurses. They explored ways to integrate study findings into daily care delivery.

The Development Phase of Transition: Mission of Nursing Explored

To further the development of the PAC, a group of nurses in the clinic conducted informal discussions about individual encounters with patients. They challenged one another to more fully explore what each experience meant to the patient and to themselves as nurses providing care. As a result of these discussions, the nurses became more aware that a shift was beginning to occur in their thinking. Discussions expanded to include philosophical beliefs about the nature of person, health, and illness and related this information to nursing practice.

Each nurse came to recognize restrictions and limitations in patient care associated with personal beliefs and values and made a conscious choice to change his or her perspective. Their prior views about person and disease had focused on illness as an obstacle to be overcome. As nurses began to shift from a disease model to a process model, however, they became able to understand the patient experience from the stories told. What also became clear was that the individual's life was more than the surgical intervention. By restricting all conversation to the surgical event, nurses found they were not fully coming to know their patients or what the illness experience truly meant. Rather, the postoperative preparation occurred in isolation and without an appreciation of the event in the person's life.

The Development Phase of Transition: Linking Theory to Practice

Throughout the transition period, the team leader was available to the nurses and stimulated further discussion. Often, the team leader would challenge the nurses to define the role of the nurse within the emerging environment of perioperative care. Patients continued to seek more than a cure for a disease. Indeed, many viewed their illness as a part of who they were as individuals. Sometimes, a cure for their disease was not even possible. During these times, PAC nurses came to understand the role they played as they worked to incorporate a picture of the whole of the person in the midst of major illness. The team leader began to link their discoveries to the work of Newman (1994), providing articles for them to read and discuss at team meetings.

PAC nurses came to recognize the limitations of a disease-oriented model and began exploring and discussing the possibility of a practice model that was more inclusive of the whole person. They began to appreciate the evolutionary process of personal growth and discovery that individuals might be undergoing and the role they played in facilitating it. The nurses discussed how they influenced patients' care and how "being present" during this vulnerable preoperative period helped to change the experience for patients.

As a result of mentoring, the PAC nurses began to seek out workshops on nursing theory, such as the one given at Massachusetts General Hospital in 1998 that discussed the nursing theories of Newman (1994, 1999) and Rogers (1970). In addition, some of the PAC nurses attended a class by Dolores Krieger on therapeutic touch. Others sought extended experiences in complementary healing through a weekend retreat in Pumpkin Hollow, New York. These experiences gave the PAC nurses increased exposure to new ideas about person, nursing, environment, and health. During the same period, nursing administrators were questioning the need for and future direction of the PAC. Nurses saw this inquiry as a challenge to define their contribution to healthcare outcomes in the perioperative setting. While PAC units at other hospitals were being closed to save costs, these PAC nurses began to articulate an expanded nursing contribution across perioperative care, and their work was increasingly valued by nursing administration.

The Development Phase of Transition: Creating the Environment of Care

During this phase of development, the team leader worked to strengthen the accomplishments made and to create a clinic environment that was more inviting for patients. At that time, nurses' offices were brightly lit and had no artwork or other decorations. The rooms lacked color or individual detail. The desk in each room was arranged so that the nurse sat behind it and the patient across from the desktop. Along with advocating other changes in the care environment, all of the nurses came to share a common belief that a space used to interview patients should make each person feel welcome. The team leader provided the resources needed to create an individual space for each nurse. Nurses were encouraged to decorate their own offices in a way that would make both the nurse and patients feel welcome. They used plants, small waterfalls, pictures, music, aroma, and softer lighting to enhance the office spaces and prepare for the nurse–patient encounter.

The clinic was repainted a muted gray color, recarpeted with a muted purple rug, and refurnished with softer, more comfortable chairs that matched the paint and carpeting. Sconce lighting and lamps replaced the glaring fluorescent lighting. Later, after reading nursing theory and relevant nursing literature, the PAC nurses began to link the changes made in the clinic with the creation of a caring environment. With the restructuring of the patient environment, nurses noticed that the entire experience of "being with" the patient was different. The patients often described the nurses' offices as "inviting."

They reported that although the clinic looked busy, the nurses seemed very relaxed and seemed to be encouraging them to do the same.

The Implementation Phase

Under continued mentoring by the team leader, nurses in the preadmission clinic increased their commitment to changing the way they delivered nursing care. It was apparent that a new model of practice was replacing the old paradigm of delivering nursing care in the PAC. Therefore, describing a new model of patient care was essential to future development of the PAC.

Gradually, the new changes were integrated into practice. Sometimes changes were informed by theory and nursing knowledge; at other times changes were made and then linked to theory. One of the first things that the nurses introduced into practice was therapeutic touch. This intentional action was undertaken to begin redefining the environment and increase patient relaxation. The nurses in the PAC put a stamp on the patient preadmission nursing assessment to determine the patient's desire to know more about therapeutic touch. To their surprise, approximately 40% of the patients chose to learn and experience therapeutic touch preoperatively and postoperatively. This number continued to increase as nurses became more comfortable with both the skill and the support they received from the team leader.

The PAC nurse also discovered that patients enjoyed the experience and expressed a desire to continue the relationship throughout the postoperative hospital stay. To satisfy this request, the PAC nurse conducted follow-up visits while the patient was in the hospital, and made follow-up phone calls once the patient had been discharged from the hospital. When the nurses visited the patients postoperatively on the units, they engaged in therapeutic touch or other nursing interventions such as being with the patient, or praying. PAC nurses noted the effects that their presence had on patient care and recognized that the patients were often "happy" to see a person with whom they had established a meaningful connection. Many times patients returned to the clinic after discharge to visit with the PAC nurse and to discuss the overall impact that the experience of being a patient in the PAC clinic had on their lives.

Newman (1994) discussed the need for nurses to be aware of their own pattern prior to meeting with patients. This is similar to Krieger's (1993) idea of being centered prior to offering therapeutic touch to others. The idea is grounded in Rogerian science and supports reciprocity and the mutual benefit of therapeutic touch for both the patient and the provider. Taking time to center oneself provided a challenge to the PAC nurses during the course of their workday, but they soon recognized that caring for self was a necessary component for caring for others. Watson (1996) supports this value, and nurses read and discussed Watson's work at team meetings.

Linking theory to practice was continuously observed as nurses began to see the event of surgery being merely one part of the person's story. This process was supported in the theoretical perspectives from Newman (1994) and Rogers (1970). Accepting the assumption that disease is a part of the whole (Rogers, 1970), and a manifestation of the underlying pattern of the person, nurses began to integrate theory to the practice model more consistently.

As part of the assessment protocol for each patient, the nurses used open-ended interviews to encourage patients to tell their stories and to relate the significant people and events in their life (Newman, 1994). Newman suggested that this invitation occur in the beginning phase of a partnership between the nurse and the patient. Focusing on assessment strategies that strengthened this relationship was consistent with the nurses' philosophical beliefs that began to emerge. These beliefs reflected (1) person as an unfolding being and open energy system, (2) the nurse as the one who is open to the exchange of energy, and (3) the partnership between the nurse and the patient as effective—together they have increased awareness and the ability to transcend to a higher level of consciousness.

Exemplars of Changed Practice

Two examples that reflect the change from a disease-based practice to the theory-based practice using the PNPM are provided to illustrate the experiences of both nurses and patients. The first occurred prior to the changes in the PAC environment. Here the nurse had an office, but she was still conducting interviews within a problem-focused model.

Exemplar 1

A 53-year-old woman came into the nurse's office describing how she was preparing to have a hysterectomy. The patient described no new symptoms, but did have a history of fibroid tumors, which in the past had caused heavy bleeding. This was not a current complaint for the patient. In fact, she had no physical symptoms or complaints. The patient did describe, however, how she had just recently lost her mother to cancer. The patient had cared for her mother over a two-year period. Prior to her mother's death, her father had been ill for some time and the patient had also participated in his care. The patient had described this surgery as her "turn to be taken care of," stating how she viewed her recovery as a sort of reprieve from all she had been through.

While this patient may indeed have needed the surgery, this exemplar raised many questions about the current surgery, life events, and the ethics, purpose, and meaning around seeking surgery at this time. Within a problem-focused model, the nurse knew something was not quite right about this patient's description of "my turn," but was unsure how to explore this issue further. The emphasis was on the surgery and related symptoms. This example is by no means atypical of a nurse–patient encounter in a fast-paced setting. There was no time or space to discuss the surgery, its timing, or its meaning in the person's life at that time. It did suggest that the nurse needed to explore the situation from a process-oriented perspective as suggested by Newman (1994) to uncover the whole pattern. An example of the changing practice in the PAC and a nurse–patient encounter that is within the framework of Newman's (1994) theory is provided next.

Exemplar 2

A 37-year-old woman again presented with uterine fibroids. The nurse welcomed her into a patient-focused setting. The nurse and the patient then talked about the significant people and events as suggested by Newman (1994). In doing so, the nurse discovered that the patient had played piano in the past and was actually quite good. The patient had given up the piano because her family thought that it was a nice hobby, but not something the patient should continue to pursue because she would not make enough money doing so. The patient shifted to a business career and was now married with children. She had no time for the piano she loved. She said sitting at her desk worsened her pelvic discomfort. Somehow this area of discomfort struck the nurse. She stated, "It was like she was pointing to this area of congestion, stifling her, and this desk job being a source for blocking a creative flow." The nurse shared these thoughts with the patient. The patient began to weep, stating that this was exactly how she felt. Together, the nurse and the patient discussed ways to bring creativity back into her life for a fuller, more complete healing that could be incorporated into her surgical recovery time and beyond.

Continuous Evaluation of the Model

The PNPM was developed and implemented over a period of two years. Adoption of the model was gradual and remains ongoing. As changes were implemented in the practice setting, the staff came to recognize that there was no returning to the previous way care was delivered. To sustain this change required much support and mentoring by the team leader, not because nurses did not want to change their practice, but rather because the change was so different from the previous practice model. Many of the nurses described the change as an inner awareness that at times created personal discomfort. Even though they had freedom to practice within a HEC-based framework and redefine nursing practice away from a medical problem orientation and toward a process model, nurses who once felt they were "experts" in a more technical role now felt vulnerable. Open-ended, process-oriented nursing allowed freedom, but was uncomfortable at first because the nurses were unsure "what would happen if" the patient asked what they were doing or why.

A second source of the discomfort was related to the nurses being truly open and authentic with the patients. As patients began to share their stories and personal vulnerabilities, the nurses began to recognize that a mutual process was emerging. Often the nurses came to recognize that the experience of "being with" the patient caused them to see themselves in a new way. They realized that they, too, were changing as individuals. The nurses frequently share personal experiences of "being with" a patient with the team leader. This exchange required time for debriefing and reflection during the work period and beyond.

Occasionally, the PAC nurses would express anger at the team leader, feeling it would be easier to just be the "expert" nurse giving out advice rather than have to change everything that had been comfortable for them. Sometimes, a nurse manifested behaviors that exhibited anger but, when discussed further, were revealed to be expressions of confusion and doubt. Each nurse required continued reinforcement and encouragement, validating the delivery of excellent nursing care even though it was different than what had been delivered under the prior model.

To cope with responses from the nurses, the team leader mentored and discussed issues with staff regularly. Following meetings with the patients, either in the clinic or on the floor, the nurses would share personal experiences with the team leader. Often, they were exuberant about the freedom "to be a nurse." They believed they were making an impact on the lives of the patients and their families as they conducted practice in this evolving model of care. The nurses were amazed with the process of "coming to know" patients more authentically, and they were surprised about how ready patients were to share their stories.

Nurses validated their beliefs about patient care with the patients. When patients would stop by the clinic following discharge to talk about their perioperative experience, they would often describe personal evolving life changes and new opportunities that had emerged since the first preoperative meeting with the nurse.

During implementation of the PNPM, nurses did not always recognize the importance of caring for self. Often, they would not permit themselves to take time to reflect during the course of the day. To address this issue, the team leader suggested that, as a group or as individuals, the nurses pray, meditate, or do therapeutic touch with one another to relieve stress and enhance feelings of self-worth. While this exercise was never time-consuming, the nurses often felt the team leader might consider this "slacking off." It was important that the team leader provided much reinforcement for the nurses and supported opportunities for nurses to care for themselves so they could care for others.

Conclusions

Creating an environment of care grounded in a nursing practice model is an ongoing process that requires vision, nursing leadership, commitment, and mentoring. Often, as problems arise in the clinical setting, nurses recognize the call for change. Leadership and guidance grounded within the ontological and philosophical roots of nursing are required to promote transformational change and improve practice. Inherent in the process of developing nursing theory-based models of care is the evolving process of personal and professional growth of the staff. Nurses practicing within a theory-based model need to identify, reflect upon, acknowledge, endorse, and practice the guiding principles and assumptions related to the discipline. As a part of the entire process related to the growth of the discipline of nursing, systematic evaluation of the practice related to outcomes for both nurse and patient is essential.

References

Flanagan, J. (2002). *Nurse and patient perceptions of the Pre-admission Nursing Practice Model: Linking theory to practice*. Dissertation Abstracts International 56 (UMI No. 30-53657).

Gordon, M. (1997). Implications for clinical reasoning and judgment. In: D. Jones & C. Roy (Eds.), *Proceedings of the Knowledge Conference 1996*. Chestnut Hill, MA: Boston College Press.

Jones, D., Coakley, A., & Flanagan, J. (1999). Nursing diagnosis at 24 and 72 hours following same day surgery with general anesthesia. In: M. Rantz & P. LeMore (Eds.), *Proceedings of the 13th North American Nursing Diagnosis* (pp. 471–477). Glendale, CA: CNAHL Information Systems.

Jones, D., Coakley, A., Dauphinee, J., & Fernesbner, W. (1998). Patient response to same day surgery with local anesthesia. AORN *Final Grant Report—AORN*.

Krieger, D. (1993). *Accepting your power to heal: The personal practice of therapeutic touch*. Santa Fe, NM: Bear and Company.

Newman, M. A. (1994). *Health as expanding consciousness* (2nd ed.). New York, NY: National League for Nursing.

Newman, M. A. (1999). The rhythm of relating in a paradigm of wholeness. *Image: Journal of Nursing Scholarship*, 31(3), 227–230.

North American Nursing Diagnosis Association (1999). NANDA: *Nursing diagnosis: Definitions and classification, 1999–2000*. Philadelphia, PA: North American Nursing Diagnosis Association.

Rogers, M. E. (1970). *An introduction to the theoretical basis of nursing*. Philadelphia, PA: F. A. Davis.

Watson, J. (1996). Watson's theory of transpersonal caring. In: P. Walker & B. Neuman (Eds.), *Blueprint for use of nursing models: Education, research, practice and administration* (pp. 141–184). New York, NY: National League for Nursing.

CHAPTER SIX

THE THEORY IS THE
PRACTICE: AN EXEMPLAR

VIRGINIA A. CAPASSO

On December 14, 1996, which was my birthday, I realized a true gift-the lived experience of intentionality, presencing, and mutuality with a patient. The experience was the culmination of a semester of doctoral education that was intended to shift and expand the paradigms of evolving nursing scholars. The experience illustrated for me how Newman's theory of *Health as Expanding Consciousness* embodies the practice of nursing (Newman, 1994).

The following discussion of the aspects of *nurse work* that are critical to the development of a therapeutic nurse-patient relationship leads into the centerpiece of this article: an exemplar of an elderly woman for whom illness is a transition point. Through a startling revelation, she shares a mutually transformative moment with this vascular clinical nurse specialist (CNS). A review of the core concepts of Newman's theory (Newman, 1986,1994) of health as expanding consciousness (HEC) permits an explication of the exemplar within the theoretical framework and discussion of the implications for patient care and nursing practice.

Nurse Work

Critical aspects of nurse work must be present in order for the nurse-patient relationship to be therapeutic. These aspects include intentionality, presencing, mutuality, knowing, and caring.

Intentionality connotes a deliberative process of thought or action that, in the context of this discussion, relates to being with and coming to know the patient (Appleton, 1993). *Presencing* is the ability to share or communicate one's truth at any one moment. *Mutuality* is a "connection with or understanding of another that facilitates a dynamic process of joint exchange between people" (Henson, 1994). The process of being mutual involves a sense of unfolding that is shared in common, a sense of moving toward a common goal, and a sense of satisfaction for all involved (Quinn, 1996). *Knowing* pertains to the unitary whole of the person rather than to the usual fragmented view of a symptom or disease. Nurses want to know so that they can understand the contextual experience and needs of the patient to be helpful (Appleton, 1993). *Caring* is the nurse's way of being with the patient whereby the nurse centers on the whole person from a humanistic perspective, feels compassion for the person in need and becomes personally involved in helping.

In a recent interview, Quinn (1996) reminded us that if nurses want to create a healing environment, they must remember that they *are* part of the environment. The nurses are the "most present, most impactive part of the environment" (Quinn, 1996) for their patients. Nevertheless, before nurses can become the healing energy with which patients interact, the nurses must first do some work on their own. They have to become healed. The first step is to *center*; that is, they have to be conscious of their impact within the patient's environment, understanding that they are *it* for the patient at that time. Out of that awareness, nurses can begin to work with their own energy to "get in touch with [one's] own pattern" (Newman, 1994).

According to Schubert (1989) a working relationship evolves in the setting of mutual connectedness of the nurse and the client, a union based on knowing each other and on trusting the part of the client. The relationship then progresses from trusting to joining to bonding.

Exemplar

On a Thursday afternoon in December, a home health nurse called and asked if I would make a consultative home visit to an elderly woman who she had been following for 4 months for slow-healing venous stasis ulcers of the lower extremities. The nurse wanted a second opinion about the status of the ulcers and the wound care regimen, which currently involved twice daily wet-to-dry normal saline dressing changes. The nurse informed me that the patient (Mrs. T.) was almost 90 years old and had been a recluse for 25 years. She only left her home-an assisted living facility-to go to the hospital because her venous stasis ulcers were so bad that she could not walk any more. Mrs. T. was deferring follow-up with her physicians until after the holidays. Although I agreed to see her the next day (Friday), my 6-year old son had the flu, which prevented my visit. I rescheduled for Saturday morning. On the way to the facility, I was consciously aware of the need to connect with this patient.

About 8 A.M. I arrived at Mrs. T.'s respite unit. Mrs. T. had been served breakfast, so we chatted while she finished eating. Discussion of my son's illness led to dialogue about the large number of people who were being admitted to the hospital for the flu. The conversation prompted her recollections of the flu epidemic of 1918. Her most striking memory was of the wagons rumbling up the street. The driver would yell, "Bring out your dead." Then, he would transport the bodies to the cemetery for burial.

During the discussion, Mrs. T. described her social and medical history to me. She told me that she had been raised by a paternal aunt and uncle after she had been given up for adoption by her divorced mother. She cared for her adoptive parents until they died at advanced ages while she continued to work for the investment division of an insurance company. During menopause, she had suffered from depression requiring hospitalization for deep analysis. She married in her 60s, but her husband died after only 3 years of marriage. After her husband's death, she was confronted with the reality of his previous divorce settlement, which made his first wife beneficiary on all of his insurance policies. In addition, she shared stories about neighbors and friends to whom she had opened her home for extended periods during times of need but from whom she is now estranged. She then confirmed that during the past 25 years, she had been a recluse. She depended on a neighbor to do her shopping every week.

About one and a half hours into a two and a half-hour visit, a look of anguish crossed Mrs. T. face. She put her hand to her mouth and said, "I don't know why, but I feel like telling you something that I've avoided telling anyone ... even in deep analysis. My adoptive father sexually abused me until I was nine years old."

She started to sob. Feeling quite shocked and unprepared for this revelation, I simply went over and hugged her while she cried. After a fairly long period of time, she composed herself and actually apologized for so unexpectedly sharing this secret with me. I told her that it was an honor and a privilege for her to trust me enough to free herself of her deepest secret. I offered that, if she were interested, we could explore the services of some very fine therapists with whom she could talk further to continue her work of healing. Then, I began her wound care.

When I removed the dressings from her lower extremities, I noted that she had almost incompressible edema of her legs below the knees. The tissue looked healthy and the drainage suggested swelling more than infection. We talked about her need to elevate her legs two to three times a day and throughout the night to decrease the swelling in her legs. We also discussed the need for follow-up with her vascular surgeon. She assured me that she would make an appointment. We made a plan for my next visit, and I departed.

I returned to see Mrs. T. one week later. When I removed the dressings, I was astounded to see the obvious improvement in Mrs. T.'s legs. There was marked reduction in her leg swelling. The depth of the ulcers also had decreased about 50% in 1 week. When asked, Mrs. T. reported that she continued to sleep on the sofa in the living room with her legs up on a chair at night but she had tried to elevate her legs more during the day. When I exclaimed about the progress that had been made in healing her leg ulcers, she said, "You know, you really helped me last week."

Health as Expanding Consciousness

This exemplar illustrates that health is much more than the absence of disease. According to Newman's theory of *Health as Expanding Consciousness*, (Newman, 1994, 1986) health and illness are rhythmic fluctuations of a single life process, in which health is the "pattern [or essence] of the whole" individual, which is defined as the interaction of the human system with the environmental system.

Consciousness is viewed as a process that is continuously evolving to a higher level (Bentov, 1978). Thus, pattern and movement are two of the major constructs of the theory. Furthermore, pattern of movement and pattern recognition are important manifestations of expanding consciousness. Prigione's (Newman, 1984) theory of dissipative structures, which is visually depicted in Figure 6.1, illustrates the pattern of movement in the evolution of consciousness.

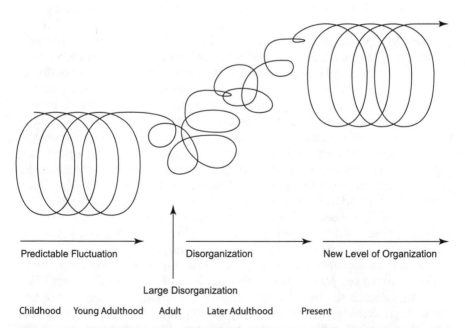

Figure 6.1.   Prigogine's theory of dissipative structures (Newman, 1994). Reprinted with permission.

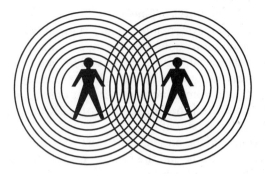

Figure 6.2. A holographic model of two-person interaction (Newman, 1994). Reprinted with permission.

The system operates in a rhythmic, predictable fashion for a while until a chance element, some critical event, brings about a giant fluctuation that propels the system into disorganized, unpredictable fluctuations, from which the system will eventually emerge at a higher level of organization (Newman, 1994).

The rhythm of movement is an integrating experience. Disease or trauma alter the natural tempo of the rhythmic pattern of movement, creating chaos (giant fluctuation) and changing cycles of receptivity.

In this relational paradigm of health, nursing intervention often occurs at a time of chaos when people are in situations they do not know how to handle (choice point). The nurse and patient enter into a partnership, "trusting that in the process of its unfolding, both will emerge at a higher level of consciousness"(Newman, 1986). The relationship can be depicted by a holographic model in which interference waves result from the interaction of energy between people in the relationship (See Figure 6.2). Pattern recognition occurs when the nurse gains insight into his or her own pattern and then the pattern of those with whom he or she is interacting. The latter requires that the nurse be fully present. Appropriate nursing action becomes apparent only as the pattern becomes apparent. The action emerges from the "truth" discovered as clients find the center of their truth and discover new rules that apply to their situations. When the insight occurs, no matter how complex the situation, the solution is simple. Pattern recognition and subsequent action constitute the transformative moment.

Analysis of the Exemplar

The exemplar describes an elderly woman who, after 25 years of seclusion, emerges from her home for treatment of severely disabling venous stasis ulcers. From the perspective of the theory of *Health as Expanding Consciousness*

(Newman, 1994, 1986), the physical illness (venous stasis ulcers) is "the critical event ... that propels [her] system into [chaos]" and, subsequently, transition.

The need for consultation about wound care permits an encounter and the development of a relationship between the patient and the vascular CNS. As a result of the information shared by the patient's primary home care nurse, the CNS is aware of the patient's previous patterns of social isolation and non-compliance with prescribed therapies. Thus, the CNS has an intentionality about presencing with the patient.

The interpenetration of the patient's and the CNS's energy fields allows the patient to discover her "truth" and the new set of rules that apply to her situation. That is, recollections of the flu epidemic of 1918 resurrect memories of the most grievous insults to the patient's health-abandonment by her mother and sexual abuse as a child. Revelation of a lifelong pattern of disconnection, distrust, and pain follows.

The memory of sexual abuse emerges in the context of a society that now acknowledges the atrocity of sexual abuse of children, punishes pedophiles, and accepts and supports victims of sexual abuse. The memory is shared in the context of an environment in which the CNS builds rapport through caring, honesty, and support. The CNS assists the patient in releasing both the emotional attachments and her need for control, thus, creating an attitude of hope and surrender (Mentgen, 1996).

The surrender of the "secret" of sexual abuse as a child is the transformative event for the patient. The revelation releases blocked energy that has been beyond her conscious awareness and underlying her history of physical and psychiatric illness (Moss, 1981). With the elimination of tension and blocked energy, energy repatterning to wholeness is possible. The decrease in the size of the patient's ulcers provides evidence of her body's rebuilding itself (Newman, 1994) and the mind-body connection in healing (Upledger, 1989).

The revelation of the "secret" is also a transformative event for the CNS. The clinical encounter actualizes the tenet that *the theory is the practice*. That is, the CNS truly realizes the experience of being fully present with a patient and coming to know the whole person through the window of an illness. The CNS becomes a healer rather than a broker of prescriptive care. The experience is almost spiritual-the embodiment of an advanced practice *nurse* rather than a physician-substitute.

Implications

The CNS has created a safe place for the patient to be vulnerable. An ongoing relationship between the CNS and the patient could help the patient to further explore patterns of interaction in her life and, potentially, transform and transcend her lifelong pattern of trauma and disconnection. The CNS may offer healing techniques, such as therapeutic touch, to help this patient center and heal herself.

If the patient chooses to be healed, the CNS may collaborate with the primary home care nurse to facilitate further a path to healing by recommending therapists with whom the patient can talk. The CNS and the home care nurse even may arrange appointments, if the patient desires; however, if the patient is not ready to talk with others, the most appropriate care may be to simply create an accepting and nonjudgmental environment in which the patient's privacy and safety are assured. Over time, the status of the patient's wound healing or her development of new ulcers may serve as indicators of her level of emotional distress.

At the institutional or professional level, the adoption of a Newman model would revolutionize nursing practice. Emphasis would shift from efficient completion of tasks to centering and presencing with patients to really come to know whole person. Newman's methodology for pattern recognition could be adopted as the format for the nursing assessment. The real source of an illness could unfold. Then, nursing care truly could be customized and have a higher likelihood of effectiveness, that is, moving the patient to a higher level of consciousness.

Summary

When the theory of *Health as Expanding Consciousness* (Newman, 1994, 1986) is the practice of nursing, the implications are clear. At the choice point when a sudden disorganizing event like an illness creates an opportunity for a nurse-patient relationship, the nurse's intentionality, presencing, and caring for the whole person promotes interpenetration of energy fields, pattern recognition, and revelation of "truths." The revelation of truths is a mutually transformative event for the nurse and the patient. The patient begins to see personal patterns of relatedness, often dating back to childhood. The recognition and acceptance of the patterns by the patient are the first steps to healing. The transformative event for the nurse is personal recognition of the power of *her presence* in helping a patient to *heal*, rather than assisting other care providers to *cure*.

Acknowledgments

The author gratefully acknowledges Dorothy Jones, Ed.D., R.N.C. (Professor and doctoral faculty, Boston College, Chestnut Hill, MA), who has shifted and expanded the author's paradigm from curing to healing; fellow doctoral students, especially Amanda Bullette Coakley, Ph.D., R.N., and Ellen Long-Middleton, Ph.D. R.N., C.S.-F.N.P., for their consultation on this manuscript;

and Debra Burke, M.S.N., M.B.A., R.N., (Nurse Manager, Vascular Nursing and Vascular Home Care Program, Massachusetts General Hospital, Boston, MA), for her nomination for this exemplar award, support for doctoral education, and colleagueship in revolutionizing nursing practice and patient care.

References

Appleton, C. (1993). The art of nursing: The experience of patients and nurses. *Journal of Advanced Nursing, 18*, 892–899.

Bentov, I. (1978). *Stalking the wild pendulum.* New York, NY: E. P. Dutton.

Henson, R.H. (1997). Analysis of the concept of mutuality. *Image: The Journal of Nursing Scholarship, 29*, 77–81.

Mentgen, J. (1992). The clinical practice of healing touch. In: D. Hover-Kramer (Ed). *Healing touch* (pp. 155–165). Albany, NY: Delmar Publishers.

Moss, R.(1981). *The I that is we.* Millbrae: Celestial Arts.

Newman, M.A. (1994). *Health as expanding consciousness* (2nd ed.). St. Louis, MO: Mosby.

Newman, M.A. (1986). *Health as expanding consciousness.* St. Louis, MO: Mosby.

Quinn, J. (1996). Therapeutic touch and a healing way. *Alternative Therapies, 2*, 69–75.

Schubert, P.E. (1989). *Mutual connectedness: Holistic practice under varying conditions of intimacy.* Unpublished doctoral dissertation. University of California, San Francisco.

Upledger, J. E. (1989). Self-discovery and self-healing. In R. Carlson & B. Shield (Eds). *Healers on Healing* (pp.67–72). New York, NY: Putnam.

CHAPTER SEVEN

THE NURSING PRAXIS OF FAMILY HEALTH

MERIAN LITCHFIELD

Introduction

My research has evolved with a focus on the nature of the relational process that gives expression to health as expanding consciousness in nursing practice with families. The meaning of health for family and nurse takes shape within the unfolding relationship that exists between them. This relational process is framed as family health and presented as nursing praxis.

Nursing Praxis

Inspired by Newman's HEC theory, the praxis relies on the premise that theory, research, and practice are one process. The researcher is as if the practitioner and, with the family, is informed by the insights that emerge through the nurse–family relationship. Through the praxis all those participating move on in new ways within their respective worlds.

Through exploration of health as expanding consciousness with families experiencing complex health circumstances, I described praxis as the interrelationship of four themes: partnership, dialogue, pattern recognition, and 'health' (its meaning). The nursing encounter with families is a partnership with the adult members. Within the partnership the dialogue evolves, enfolding all that transpires between nurse and family and unfolding through revelations of how happenings and situations are interconnected. At a point in time, it becomes clear to the nurse that the people have gained insight into their circumstances and how they might move on in life, accommodating disease, disability, and treatments in a new way. In retrospect, through reflecting on the entire dialogue, the nurse can see this movement as a process of recognizing pattern. As participants, the family and nurse have together found order inherent in the chaos of family life. "Health" has acquired particular meaning for both the family and the nurse. The nurse can then reflect on participation in the partnership to examine the values that have shaped it. I present this process as practice wisdom (Litchfield, 1999).

Vision and community are core values. They are embedded in my personal and professional life, and resonant with the philosophical foundations of Newman's theory. *Vision* refers to an extended view across place and time into the past and future, to give meaning to the health experience in the here and now. *Community* refers to a sense of connectedness and human belonging as family, friend, and citizen, of love and caring. These values underpin the premises of the participatory paradigm for the praxis; that is, in our interrelatedness, we are the creators of our worlds and on a quest for meaning, seeking pattern as order in chaos. Within this paradigm, research takes the form of practice and its methodology is a "dynamic, mutual process of expanding consciousness" (Newman, 1995, p. 103). As such, it expresses the wholistic focus of the discipline: "caring in the human health experience" (Newman, Sime & Corcoran-Perry, 1991). Through the dialogue, evolving toward insight as action, the health experience in the context of life and living takes narrative form, expressing the meaning of family health. In Figure 7.1, the themes of this praxis process are represented as the facets of a tetrahedron to depict their interrelationship.

Exemplar

An exemplar of this research-as-if-practice encounter with one family provides an illustration of the praxis. The abstracted family predicament introduces the narrative. It is followed by the methodology through which the health experience was elicited from the parents and took its narrative form for presentation. The ending of the narrative is framed in a statement of outcome. To conclude, reflection on the meaning of family health reveals theoretical significance of the nursing praxis as expression of expanding consciousness.

The Family Predicament

I first made contact with the family in the pediatric unit of the hospital. At two years of age, Ben had been admitted yet again with a severe acute exacerbation of his asthma and was being stabilized on a new medication regime. Ben's hospitalizations had become almost habitual, occurring every one to two

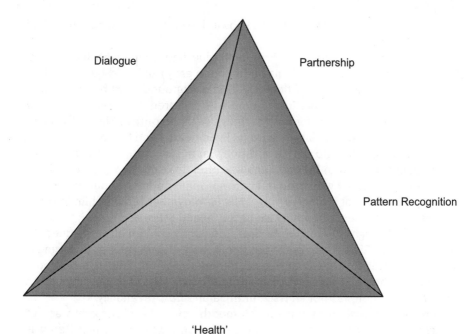

Figure 7.1.   The process of praxis.

months. Each time the treatment plan had been revised, and often a new drug had been introduced into his care regimen. His mother, Sarah, was trying to think positively, to believe that this time, with the plans for monitoring by medical and nursing practitioners, along with the revised prescription of steroid treatment and the new trial medication, she would have the key to controlling his condition.

During his acute hospitalizations, Sarah stayed in the hospital unit with Ben, while his father Tana remained at home looking after three-year-old Simon. Sarah said while Ben was at home she tried hard to do what she had been taught about controlling the predisposing environmental factors and adhering to the medication regimen. But, they always ended up in the hospital regardless of their efforts. Sarah was grateful to the specialist community nurse who visited the home sometimes. The nurse helped her use and check the equipment and was very encouraging.

The pediatric staff in the hospital felt frustrated they had not been able to control Ben's disease. They were skeptical about what was happening at home after Ben was discharged, wondering if Sarah really was fully compliant with the treatment instructions. Despite their interventions, nothing had prevented Ben's rehospitalizations in an acute state. Sarah had kept all the clinic appointments. The visiting specialist nurse felt Sarah knew what was required and was a committed mother, although needing support and reassurance.

None of the health professionals had knowledge of the tension and turmoil of everyday life in the home.

The path of increasing turmoil in family life had begun with Ben's birth. Before this, life for Sarah and Tana hadn't been easy but it had been relatively orderly. They came from different ethnic backgrounds and had worked at their relationship preparing for a home with children. Culturally, parenting had particular significance for both partners. With the birth of Simon, they had settled into family living. Sarah's parents lived nearby and looked after Simon from time to time to help out. In addition, Sarah saw quite a lot of her sister and kept in contact with friends. Tana was often in contact by phone with his large extended family who lived out of town, some out of the country. He was working, although for a meager wage. His employment brought him into the cliques of workmates, but otherwise he socialized little.

With Sarah's tight rein on the budget, the family could make ends meet financially. After Simon was born, the family had qualified for a government housing assistance benefit and paid minimal rent for their two-bedroom apartment. They had no car. The apartment block was on a major bus route and transportation was not an issue until Sarah's next pregnancy.

Ben was born when Simon was 16 months old. The pregnancy was not straightforward, and the birth was protracted and difficult. At first Ben was sleepy, like a "floppy doll." He did not cry, and Sarah had to find ways to persuade him to get him to feed. She thought it strange that he should be so different from Simon but the pediatrician, community physician, and nurses said all appeared normal. Back home, however, family life began to disintegrate into chaos.

When Ben was a few weeks old, Tana found him blue, cold, and scarcely breathing. He was resuscitated in the ambulance. From then on, Sarah and Tana were frightened of his condition. Sarah particularly was constantly alert to his breathing, monitoring him day and night. Ben had repeated severe bouts of breathlessness with chest infections for which he was hospitalized, and eventually given a diagnosis of asthma.

Sarah's parents moved to a different part of the country so Tana began to take time off from work to look after Simon while Sarah tended to Ben. This led to tension with his employer and eventually, when Tana's leave entitlement ran out, he lost his job. Over the next two years, this chaos played out as a complex series of events and strained relationships. While the most pivotal of the health problems in family life was Ben's respiratory disease and its management, both Sarah and Tana also had episodes of hospitalization, fortunately brief, with acute, seemingly unrelated pathologies. Their treatments were eventually successful in curing and controlling the problems, but without attention being given to the complexity of all that was going on at home, the mounting strain was aggravated.

The family became divided. Ben had his mother's attention almost continuously: "He always wants his mother." In competition, three-year-old Simon became hyperactive and aggressively demanding, and he slept erratically. Tana focused his attention on his elder son: "He's Dad's boy." Nights were disturbed. To manage Ben's two-hourly treatment regimen and required monitoring throughout the night, Sarah shared the bedroom with Ben; Tana shared the second bedroom with Simon.

During the day, life went in different directions as well. The parents knew that leaving the house exposed Ben to many environmental factors that could exacerbate Ben's asthma, so one parent always stayed home with him. As Ben grew into toddlerhood, he became hyperactive too, a condition attributed to the doses of steroid medication he received. In addition, the treatments fostered a ferocious appetite, so he was constantly searching for food, he ate anything he could find. Shopping, a time of stress for Sarah, had to be done twice a week, instead of once. Daily, when they were together, the two toddlers were either fighting or destroying things. They were separated, with a parent managing each, as much as possible. The parents did not go out together, nor did the family as a whole, and they scarcely talked.

There was a spiral of increasing financial hardship. To ease the strain, Simon was enrolled in a childcare center three days a week. During this time, a behavioral therapist became involved in his care. Sarah then took other people's children into the home to earn the money to pay for Ben's therapy. But this strategy was not a dependable source of income, because of Ben's hospitalizations. The hospitalizations were free, but their associated costs mounted. Sarah stayed in the unit with Ben, and Tana took Simon to visit in the evenings and had to purchase a meal at the restaurant. When Ben was at home, the multiple visits to the clinic incurred fees. In the clinic, the nurse and the physician monitored Ben's condition and continued to administer some of the treatments. The visits increased to daily, sometimes twice daily, when Ben's condition was found to be deteriorating. There were additional regular visits to specialists. With a sick child, and sometimes unwell parents, the family had to rely on taxis for transportation. They survived financially on a range of government benefits.

Movement outside the home became increasingly restricted and the family was financially strapped. Their social contacts collapsed. Tana's phone calls to his family became unaffordable. Sarah could not keep up with her friends. Her sister had a child who was also repeatedly hospitalized with asthma, and both were too preoccupied to get together. Thus time and circumstances collapsed the family's personal and social worlds— and no one else knew. The parents were constantly tired but went on struggling, just to get through each day. Their life was like being on a treadmill. They could not imagine how life could be different and feared for their children's future.

This was the predicament when we met. It was through the praxis methodology that the predicament became known in its complexity.

Praxis Methodology

Nurses in the hospital pediatric unit referred the family to my project. I was interested in how we might develop nursing practice for families with children who were repeatedly hospitalized. Sarah consented to my proposed series of approximately weekly visits to the home to talk about the family's experience with repeated hospitalizations. During my four visits to their home, different storylines unfolded and became interwoven, and the narrative of their life took its form as my professional project. A fifth visit a year later was for practical reasons of consent for publication of the narrative but also contributed to the praxis.

Dialogue

My role (researcher as if practitioner) in this praxis is to participate openly in dialogue with the family members, to work at understanding what is going on for them in relation to health and family life. I have no preset questions, guidelines for my role, or theoretical framework to prompt data collection. Through my exploration of the theory of health as expanding consciousness in a unitary, transformative paradigm, I have become comfortable with the idea of an evolving, participatory method, for practice as well as for research. My title of nurse and researcher, essential for me to introduce myself, does suggest certain expectations but these just merge into our dialogue. It is an unaffected conversation that can evolve in its own way, simply because of who we all are as participants in it. We all have our own stories to tell that are fully and equally important although this dialogue is unreservedly focused on understanding the family's predicament. I ask questions spontaneously and pursue topics when I think they are important to the family. Everything said—and what is unsaid—is relevant, as is how it is said.

Only Sarah was present on my first two visits to the home. She agreed to my use of a tape recorder to prompt memory later. At the beginning, the dialogue was restrained and formal, just as it is when strangers meet. Sarah explained Ben's most recent hospitalization, the admission procedure, and the treatment plan. To elaborate, she delivered a timeline of events from Ben's pregnancy through birth and the sequence of investigations, diagnosis, and treatment plans. But I wanted to know more than this if we were to go beyond what was already happening.

I have found in my praxis research that, after an episode of particularly intense storytelling, it is helpful to me to put what I have heard into my own words. This sets us off again on another tack of elucidation. The stories become complex. I wonder, with growing respect, how people manage to live in such complexity and chaos. But gradually, as we move circuitously through time and place, I can see threads in family life emerging. I have learned to ignore the urge to analyze what I am hearing, to frame any one of the storylines according to any of the plethora of theories I have studied in class. I have learned to allow myself to be absorbed into the dialogue, to become lost in it and emotionally moved by the family's experience. I have learned to resist the temptation to close the partnership prematurely, when I think I know, or to withdraw when the circumstances seem too chaotic to ever reach any understanding. I know now that order does emerge, that storylines do become coherent, and that they can eventually take the form of a narrative: Pattern recognition takes its own time and course.

On my third visit, Tana joined us for the first time. English was not his first language, and he was reticent in replying when questions were posed directly to him. I did not push him to talk, but he was intensely interested as Sarah and I continued. At the end of this third visit, I felt my rapport with Sarah was such that I was ready to write an overview of the family's health circumstances to be given to the couple to read. When I returned on the subsequent visit, they had seemingly devoured its every word.

In this interim text I write storylines, still raw, interweaving my summary statements with direct quotes from the audiotape transcript when I have one. Even without audiotaping, the voices of the family members readily come to mind as I write. The purpose of this written text in the praxis partnership is not to check out the accuracy of my understanding or the adequacy of my description; I do not seek affirmation or corrections. Rather, the text is information for the family participants regarding how I understand their situation. Of course, it reveals a lot about who I am, and about my values and interests that underpinned what I attended to. Thus all participants contribute who we are as human beings, and we all move to see circumstances with greater abstraction as we reflect on the dialogue. This is the in-forming capacity of the dialogue, an expression of expanding consciousness in Newman's theory.

Insight

When I arrived for my fourth visit, it was, unexpectedly, Tana who met me at the door. He was waiting to talk. The text had spurred the couple to sit and talk together. Now they sat side by side talking with considerable animation—yet poignancy—about what they saw as their family circumstances. They discussed how the predicament had arisen and what they would be doing about it: "It is very sad, the way he has been and how we coped. We didn't know it was very bad . . . he had such a rough time because we just went from month to month (repeated hospitalizations) . . . you forget what he was like in the beginning, when he was born—and what we went through when he was younger . . . to think about (all that has happened) again, exactly how it was—when you see it in black and white (the summary text)."

Specifically, in the context of all that had transpired, Sarah and Tana had together resolved that they would get Ben off his medication by the time he reached school age. They had identified his medication as the key factor in their family predicament—its impact on him and the administration regimen on the family as a whole. This focused our conversation. With this insight, I could clarify the storyline threads unfolding through the dialogue. The interrelationships between and among these elements began to make sense to me. The couple was already beginning to address the issues. The natural ending of our partnership was approaching.

The insight is recognizable as a statement of action, where action concerns how people will get on with life and living, how the change expresses their vision of health circumstances. It is not the reiteration of anything written in the interim text; it is novel for all participants. The change could not have been proposed earlier, or even imagined, but once mentioned, the significance is obvious. I have a sense of its meaning for the family because I have participated in their story-telling. I share with them in the excitement of the moment when we realize how life can be different.

The conversation that followed was easy, as it roved around the insight and implications. The revelation of the division of the family had been sobering because each parent had a clear sense of parenting role and responsibility. A change in Tana's interaction with his younger son was immediately apparent: "I treat them (the two boys) just the same now." Sarah, seeing herself as having a pivotal role in family development, had recognized that what they had achieved would be the essential foundation of confidence for subsequent efforts: "It was good . . . we had to do it together . . . you just have to depend on your own . . . I have to cope on my own."

Sarah had obtained information from the library about Ben's latest medication. With an increased understanding of the medication and its side effects, the parents could assume the management of the treatment plan themselves instead of constantly visiting the clinic. They were confident in their ability to judge when Ben was heading into exacerbation and be more responsive and timely with treatments: "I used to sit back and take it, but you get to know what he needs and what he is on (medication) and you are the one living with him . . . if I don't think he needs as much medicine, I won't give it to him." Sarah and Tana told the specialist they would not agree to further experimenting with any more new medications: "The doctors will prescribe stuff, but they are not living with him. It's easy for (the specialist) to say 'pump in the (medication),' but he is not up with him all night, every night." The parents knew what support they wanted from health professionals, and now they would manage it.

Eventually the conversation reached a natural end, when there was no more to be said. Later, I tidied the summary text and delivered it to the couple as my point of closure. A year after this encounter, our conversation picked up again just where we had left it, with the same warmth and animation as it is with friends. We caught up on the year's activities. There was no interest in talking more about the turmoil surrounding Ben's early life. The experience of our partnership was well past and not noteworthy now, a mere moment in the unfolding pattern of family life. The family had moved on in their life, and they had done it in their own way together.

I did have an opportunity to see how the parents' resolve to get Ben off medication had played out since the ending of our partnership. Ben had not been back to hospital. He still experienced symptoms such as wheezing, but the family was now involved in activities just like other families. Roles had changed. Sarah was employed, and Tana was the children's caregiver during the day. Sarah's income had enabled them to buy a car. The management of the boys' behavior was no longer of note. Sarah and her sister collaborated in child care. These activities seemed banal—but I knew the deeply transformative significance for this family.

Throughout my research I have understood a family's statement of insight to be affording me a window into their world. Within the context of the family predicament their abstraction becomes insight for me, and my horizon expands to incorporate more diversity and complexity in the meaning of health and nursing. For the family and for me, as if practitioner, the meaning that surfaces during the dialogue plays out in our respective worlds. Families are pleased to be getting on with life and living, to have passed "the bad patch." As a researcher, I present family health as a narrative of the predicament, the process of praxis in relation to outcome, and its theoretical significance as an expression of health as expanding consciousness.

Outcome

The practitioner with a praxis approach has achieved the health outcome by reaching an ending to the partnership and articulating the meaning of health as the process of change in people's lives. As exemplified in this story, through praxis the two parents came to see how the efforts to treat and control Ben's respiratory disease had paradoxically controlled the extent to which they could, as a family, live with and manage it. They had been caught in the immediacy and repetitiveness of their efforts and had been devastated by their impotence. The partnership had given them the opportunity to gain insight through which they reconstructed their life as a whole family and moved past the time of turmoil and strife. In becoming informed, self-directive, and assertive, they avoided the disruption of further hospitalization with Ben. They moved on with their lives with a facility and prospects none of us could have imagined previously.

Family Health

The exemplar presents the meaning of family health for one family as it evolved through the caring dialogic process to be given form as a narrative by the nurse. Action inherent in the insight was manifested as change in the life of the family. This change was integral to the partnership and was a transformative process. At the outset, the family predicament of chaos and strife had centered on the treatment of the child's diagnosed disease. Through the praxis, the family came to understand and know how to live with the disease process in a new way, accommodating it into their everyday activities, and they shifted the meaning of family health to a process of expanding consciousness.

The importance of family health viewed as a process in this way lies in the belief that change is creative and involves choice. The narrative we can present of family health expresses how people gain a view of the future and a sense of community. The participation of the nurse is essential. For the nurse undertaking praxis, pattern recognition is a novel process, unique to each partnership and providing the opportunity to reflect, to challenge existing knowledge, to examine personal values, and to validate and evolve theories.

Conclusion

To be consistent with the theoretical premises, this exemplar is presented as an illustration rather than a blueprint for replication. It is an expression of my exploration and articulation of the process of praxis inspired by Newman's theory. In New Zealand, a three-year project of innovation in primary health care nursing is providing the opportunity for nurses to develop this praxis of family health in a rural nursing service scheme. Thus this praxis will continue to evolve as the process of health as expanding consciousness.

References

Litchfield, M. C. (1999). Practice wisdom. *Advances in Nursing Science*, 22(2), 62–73.

Newman, M. A. (1995). A *developing discipline*. New York, NY: National League for Nursing.

Newman, M. A., Sime, A. M., & Corcoran-Perry, S. A. (1991). The focus of the discipline of nursing. *Advances in Nursing Science*, 14(1), 1–6.

CHAPTER EIGHT

ENGAGING WITH COMMUNITIES IN A PATTERN RECOGNITION PROCESS

MARGARET DEXHEIMER PHARRIS

Introduction

The applicability and significance of Margaret Newman's theory of health as expanding consciousness (HEC) to community health nursing practice has evolved with my own practice and research over the past decade. For many years, I had used Newman's theory to guide my nursing practice with survivors of sexual assault and abuse as they incorporated the experience of victimization into their lives. Partnership with a caring nurse who practices from a HEC perspective is particularly meaningful for individuals and families during the times of disruption and disorganization brought on by violent victimization. This chapter presents the use of HEC in partnership with communities.

Relevant HEC Concepts and Community Process

From the HEC perspective, the nursing partnership with individuals and families is nonprescriptive, is noninterventionist, and involves fully open attentiveness and unconditional warm regard. The nurse does not enter into the relationship with a preset notion of what *should* happen, but rather engages in a mutual dialogue, focusing on that which is meaningful to the individual/

family, trusting that important insights will arise through the dialogue if needed. In this process, new meanings of health emerge and a widened repertoire of possible actions is realized (Jonsdottir, Litchfield & Pharris 2003; Litchfield, 1999; Newman, 1994a, 2002). The nature of a nursing partnership from this perspective is further articulated by Jonsdottir and colleagues.

My expanded view of HEC nursing research to encompass the community level took root when I was working with survivors of violence in the mid-1990s. Representatives from the city public health department approached me to join them on a team with epidemiologists and community leaders to analyze the pattern of rapidly increasing youth homicide in our community. The team met over several months. During this time, we carefully reviewed data from police, court, and economic assistance records for each young person who had committed murder. Conceptual diagrams were drawn of everything that was known about the circumstances surrounding the murders. We found that, in the end, we knew very little other than that youth homicide never occurred on Tuesday evenings in our city and that most of the murders involved firearms. In particular, we knew precious little about the youths who were incarcerated for murder or their patterns of relationships with family, friends, and the community prior to the murders.

I had just completed work using the HEC pattern recognition process with a young gang leader, who, when the process was finished, expressed deep gratitude. He indicated that he had gained much from the pattern recognition process. Both of us came away from our dialogue with new meaning and deeper insights into our lives and the nature of our relationships within the community. This young man took actions that eventually led him out of his violent lifestyle. Through this process, I came to realize that Newman's hermeneutic dialectic research methodology could also shed light on the meaning and nature of the youth homicide pattern in our community. However, I was not sure how to embark on understanding the pattern, other than knowing that it was essential to engage the incarcerated youth in the dialogue. I turned to the counsel and work of Margaret Newman (1979, 1986, 1990, 1994a, 1994b), Merian Litchfield (1999), Pat Tommet (2003), Emiko Endo (1998), Frank Lamendola (1998), and Norma Kiser-Larson (2002). Through our dialogues, and through the influence of the work of Moch (1990) and Jonsdottir (1998), I came to realize the importance of the *process* of being fully attentive to what was meaningful for the youth versus setting my sights solely on *identifying factors* that led these young people to murder. I was constantly reminded to *trust the process* and to accept that the necessary insight into the pattern of the whole would follow. This model represented a drastic paradigm shift for me—one not enthusiastically embraced by many faculty dissertation committees or clinicians, who are often locked into positivist views of how research must be conducted to "assure scientific rigor." For graduate nursing students embarking on research and attracted to the HEC perspective, such views can be a stumbling block. They are often told to specify a rigid protocol of inquiry and to classify data findings into themes, which takes them through a process that is particulate and deterministic in nature and away from an appreciation of wholeness of pattern.

HEC: The Unitary Paradigm and Praxis

From a unitary paradigm, if we are to understand the whole, we must use a methodology that does not narrow our vision. When the focus is on predetermined outcomes (e.g., finding out what *caused* the murders) and the evaluation or measurement of prescribed variables (e.g., psychiatric disorders, gang involvement), we risk losing sight of the wide range of intricate complexities of people's lives and the ways in which we are all woven together as a society. By limiting our research to causal entities and assuming they are operant, we curtail the breadth of our findings and deny the full possibility of community transformation. In addition, we negate the reality that the people involved in an experience have the best insight into their community's problems and health. We simply need to attend to the process of engaging their wisdom and insights to uncover this information.

Newman (1990) refers to her methodology as "research as praxis." Research takes on the form of practice and, at the same time, informs practice. Research, theory, and practice are reflexively engaged as an expanding whole. In a compelling review of the way the concept of praxis has been espoused by Marxist, feminist, and emancipatory critical theories, as well as by Newman (1990, 1992), Connor (1998) expands the dialogue on research as praxis and its importance for informing nursing practice and theory. She distinguishes Newman's focus on process from the view of praxis-oriented research methodology advocated from a critical social science perspective, which aims at empowerment, societal transformation, and construction of a more just society. From my experience of utilizing the HEC hermeneutic dialectic methodology at the community level, the intention to *empower* and *change* society is not consistent with a unitary paradigm, because it assumes that power is not already situated within the community and that the community needs to be acted upon.

Also, power can be understood as control rather than knowledge. Rather than backing away from social transformation, the HEC hermeneutic dialectic methodology focuses on the relational process of interpreting meaning and engaging seemingly opposing views in dialogue. It is associated with profound transformation. Each transformation is not predefined or aimed for, but rather is a construction of the process. The nurse attends to engagement and trusts that what should arise from the community will arise, knowing that power is already present. The nurse also trusts that answers to specified problems will become clear, along with the necessary actions to be taken. The nurse does not need to assume responsibility for instigating or controlling those actions (Jonsdottir, Litchfield & Pharris, 2003).

The Pattern Recognition Process for Adolescents

To explore how the concepts within Newman's HEC played out in one community's experience, let us return to the community troubled by its rising youth homicide rate, the prisons, and the youths incarcerated within them. After obtaining the human subjects' approval, I set out to apply the HEC methodology as proposed by Newman (1994) and utilized by previous Newman scholars (Endo, 1998; Endo et al., 2000; Jonsdottir, 1998; Kiser-Larson, 2002; Picard, 2000; Tommet, 2003) to engage people with a similar disease process or social situation in the pattern recognition process. I conducted a series of individual interviews with each of 12 incarcerated young men. The sessions were audiotaped and transcribed verbatim.

While any broad, open-ended question focusing on the meaning of health can be used to initiate the pattern recognition process, for me and the young men in my study, it was helpful to start out by simply asking about the most meaningful people and events in their lives. Most of the youths responded with a quizzical expression, saying something like, "Hey, aren't you a nurse? Don't you want to take my blood pressure or test me for STDs or something?" I responded by talking about the caring nature of nursing practice and presenting a wider view of health than just the absence of disease. To begin the dialogue, I asked each young man to tell me about the first important memory they had from when they were little, which quickly focused them on important relationships and events.

When I came back the second week, each person commented that he had spent many nights laying awake thinking about what was meaningful—no one had ever asked the youths that question before, nor had they systematically thought about it on their own. The second interviews were the longest and most intense. Each subsequent week we reviewed and revised a diagrammatic representation of the most important events, people, and transformation points in their lives, and each week I added what they had said to a chronological narrative. This process was repeated until they could look at the diagram and see it as depicting everything that was meaningful in their life. We then turned our attention to the narrative, making corrections, deleting sections they did not want in the final copy, and changing all identifying names and places to protect confidentiality. At our final meeting, I gave each youth a copy of the narrative, which was book length, and a copy of the diagram. At that meeting, I also asked each participant to reflect on the pattern recognition process.

In reflecting on what it was like to look at patterns of meaningful relationships and events in their lives, most of the youths made a comment like, "Aw, I wish we could have done this before I caught my case" (before I was arrested for murder). Yet that was not likely, because prior to the murders, each of them was completely cut off from meaningful relationships with pro-social adults and was using alcohol and marijuana on a daily basis. Even though they had seen a nurse in the emergency department, STD clinic, or juvenile detention facility within a month before they murdered, they recounted those visits as having been brief and focused only on physical care. When nurses have limited time and are mandated to attend to medically delegated tasks as their priority concern, partnering with patients to reflect on the meaning of their heath predicament is limited.

The pattern recognition process in the prison helped these youths see relationships for what they were and deepened their understanding of themselves and the future. One of the drawbacks of using diagrams for pattern recognition is that it locks the pattern into a fixed constellation, when what is meaningful will actually expand and change over time as new insights are reached. This was evidenced by the youths redrawing the constellations of meaningful relationships and events differently from week to week as they repatterned their lives in prison. Litchfield (1993, 1999) uses a narrative configuration of what is meaningful as health, which is less static and may be more useful, especially during adolescence when cognitive abilities are undergoing rapid change from concrete to abstract conceptualizations. However, at the time I used the pattern recognition process with the incarcerated youths, most were concrete thinkers. This seemed related to their age and the fact that many were mildly depressed immediately after incarceration. Diagrams seemed to be more helpful in engaging concrete thinkers in reflecting on what is meaningful.

The ability to think abstractly plays a role in assigning meaning to events and in envisioning motives and possible actions. In a study utilizing Newman's (1994a) pattern recognition process with young adults who have type 1 diabetes, Okhlke (2002) found that, when looking back on their adolescence, the subjects identified the point at which they were able to transition from their parents controlling their diabetes to controlling it themselves as the time when "I just grew up." They suddenly realized that they would have long-term untoward consequences of uncontrolled blood sugars; at that point, they became motivated to manage their diabetes. This seemed to be a sudden new cognitive capability. The youths incarcerated for murder experienced the same phenomenon. When the drugs, alcohol, and depression wore off and they transitioned from middle to late adolescence, they suddenly could ponder meaning and could envision a variety of outcomes on the horizon of their lives. Unfortunately, for participants in the study, they were destined to remain in prison for many years.

The majority of these youth reflected on the experience of being in jail itself as having significantly changed the way in which they were able to look at their lives. The restrictions on their movement and space related to physical confinement, and the expanded sense of time as they faced being in the same place for decades, intensified their quest for finding meaning in their experiences. This awareness is consistent with Newman's (1976, 1982) early work on the relationship between time, space, movement, and expanding consciousness. Over the weeks the patterns of movement in prison also changed—going from a uniformly tough, controlled manner to a more relaxed and uniquely individual way of moving. By the third or fourth visit, most cried as they recounted events in their life, something they had not been able to do since long before they were incarcerated. This transformation seemed to be a spiraling, dynamic process, beginning with the development of a trusting relationship in which life events could be shared and the meaning and nature of important events and relationships could be understood. Moving to the point where the young men were able to let go of the shame they had been feeling and connect to a renewed sense of themselves, they were being able to develop a more trusting relationship and go deeper into the meaning of important events and relationships (Pharris, 2002). Just as the capability to think abstractly arises during adolescence, so does the ability to feel shame, which teens do as they look back on stigmatizing and traumatic events in their lives:

> For the youth . . . shame seemed to create a distorted self-image similar to that of a circus mirror—making their negative points appear distortedly large and their positive points appear distortedly small. The process of pattern recognition shattered that distorted image and established a more realistic one. The caring nurse–participant interaction has the potential to create a pure, clear reflection pool through which the participant can see himself clearly and accurately. In this process the youth is able to see his true self and recognize his strengths (Pharris, 2002, p. 38).

This clearer vision extended to a new conceptualization of how the youths wanted to get on with their lives. By our last visit, all of them had articulated having taken actions consistent with their expanded sense of what was meaningful to them. These actions ranged from enrolling in school or work, to withdrawing from bullying, to contacting fathers and other family members who had been absent but whose importance arose in our reflective dialogue. One young man, who by the end of our time together had given up his leadership position in a gang and had entered college, explained that he found it easy to talk because I just listened and attended to what was meaningful to him. He contrasted this to the visits of a social worker friend of his mother, who came in to see him and kept asking about what his gang tattoos meant and where he had gotten his guns. In addition, he commented on how the social worker's questions were asked, which blocked any meaningful dialogue. From my personal reflections, I realized that if I had gone into the prison to persuade the young men to stop their gang involvement or to figure out where they got their guns, it would have been a much different experience yielding little insight. From the HEC perspective, the outcome cannot be anticipated at the beginning; it is understandable only in retrospect, and signifies the point where the nurse–patient partnership can draw to a close (Litchfield, 1999; Jonsdottir, Litchfield & Pharris, 2003; Newman, 1994b, 2002).

The Emerging Pattern of the Community

In comparing the life patterns of the young men, what became apparent was not a common pattern of pathologically disturbed youth, but rather a common pattern of interaction with the community that surrounded them. What arose was *our* pattern as a community. As I listened, I literally entered into several young men's stories. For example, in describing a pivotal point in his life, one young man described the pain of going with his mother at age six to the trauma center after his uncle was shot. He described being told that his uncle was dead and recounted his mother falling into the nurse's arms. As he told the story, my perspective changed from that of the six-year-old to that of the nurse. A deep sense of grief arose within me as I realized that I was the charge nurse that night in the emergency department and it was into my arms that his mother collapsed. I could vividly remember his six-year-old eyes staring at me as I attended to his mother. What I could not remember was how I responded to him afterwards—an action that took on more significance in retrospect.

The common pattern of the community surrounding these young men has been reported in depth elsewhere (Pharris, 2002). Each of the youths had experienced significant abuse and/or separation from their respective families when they were young. Later, they experienced a stigmatizing event between the ages of 9 and 12, for which they could not access the help of an adult. Soon they began skipping school and getting into trouble (e.g., stealing, fighting, setting fires). At about this time, many began having frequent casual sex with many different people. They expressed a yearning for intimacy and a place where they felt connected within the community or family. All then moved into a stage during which they used drugs and alcohol to numb their pain. In addition, they experienced feeling increasingly alienated and depressed, and no longer caring about life—their own or that of others. Soon, each obtained access to a gun. The murders they committed occurred in a way that they could just have easily been the one who was killed. The homicides had a suicidal edge. Once in jail, all resented being there, but felt it was better than being back in their chaotic and crazy existence prior to the murders.

Community Patterning

What became obvious upon comparing the patterns of the young men were the places where we as community failed to protect and engage them in a healthy way. To validate this community pattern and understand it more fully, I took the pattern I saw and stories that exemplified it to 16 community agencies and groups, ranging from community residents, to youth workers, to chaplains, policy makers, child protection workers, public health nurses, social workers, juvenile detention staff, and emergency and pediatric nurses and physicians. As I presented the pattern, each group validated the places where they could identify disconnecting from youth at risk and failing to engage these young people in meaningful ways. Each of the groups saw themselves in the young men's stories. It was an *ah-ha* experience, as all discerned the ways in which such community groups need to reweave their presence in young people's lives and in the lives of their families.

This process led me to the realization that not only can pattern recognition be used with individuals and families, but also whole communities can be engaged in the pattern recognition process. Often community health interventions are based on national or international studies and fail to take into account the unique pattern of interrelationships and historical happenings within the specific community. In addition, the strengths and insights of the people who live and work there go unnoticed.

Identifying Barriers to Health for Women and Girls of Color

In the fall of 2001, Pilot City Health Center was designated a Community Center of Excellence in Women's Health (CCoEWH) by the United States Office of Women's Health. A condition of funding was that the center develop a community-based action research plan to identify barriers to health for women and girls of color. A research team was formed that consisted of the coordinator of the CCoEWH, myself as a faculty member of the College of St. Catherine, a partner in the CCoEWH, and three graduate nursing students who willingly joined in a research process where they had no control over what the research question would be. The only criterion was that they would be engaged in a process of pattern recognition with women in the community utilizing Newman's theory of HEC. The community research process was called Community-Based Collaborative Action Research (CBCAR). This was thought to be an appropriate mnemonic, in that like a cab car or taxi, the research team was at the service of the community taking them where they wanted to go, knowing how to drive the research methodology as we traveled along together. In a conversation with Margaret Newman (personal communication, May 28, 2003), we decided that the HEC theory was like the headlights shining light on where we might go and making visible what was present when we got there.

CBCAR differed from traditional community research methodologies in that it combined the insight of the community into its own situation with the knowledge of the hermeneutic dialectic research process of college faculty and students. The process was a dialogic collaboration in which knowledge, skills, and insights were shared and transformation became a possibility for all involved. Essential elements were identified within the process and included a continued dialogue and reflection with the women's advisory council of the CCoEWH and the larger community. The goal was to discern the community pattern, with a commitment being made to seek out critical friends (community-based, theory-based, and methodology-based) to scrutinize the process and its findings. Critical friends were essential to the dialectic aspect of the research process, enhancing the understanding and validity of the process and the findings.

Initially, women from the community were invited to come and help discern the research question that would help us identify the barriers to health for women and girls of color in a community that had experienced some of the greatest health disparities in the nation. Fifty women came to the first meeting and met for four hours in large and small groups trying to discern the barriers. The women decided to return and continue the dialogue on another Saturday morning, at which time 65 women representing an array of ethnic groups reflective of the community came to participate in the dialogue. The groups broke into eight dialogue circles, and each group reported back to the larger group that they saw racism as the greatest barrier to health. Working together, a plan was developed to engage women and girls throughout the community in both focus groups and individual interviews to explore personal experiences concerning the interplay of racism, health, and well-being.

The research team met with predesignated community racism and health experts, HEC scholars, and focus-group methodology experts to critique and help shape our process. Over a several-month period, women from the community who were part of the research team joined with nursing graduate students and faculty to conduct 14 focus groups and a series of individual interviews involving women from African American churches, Hmong women, African immigrant women, Latina women, health center patients, elders, Native American women, women recruited on the street, teen peer educators, a teen support group, block club leaders, and Lao women. The team gathered the many stories from the transcribed taped interviews and stripped them of identifying information. Then women from the community were invited to join the research team for the data analysis process of identifying and drawing out the important patterns of relationships and experiences.

The group's next step was to determine how to present the emerging pattern back to the larger group of women on the advisory council. Those of us who had been involved in analyzing the data were transformed by the process of taking in the women's stories. The group came to realize that a huge gulf of disconnection and misunderstanding existed between the various ethnic groups within the community and between healthcare providers and patients. The problem was one of not being known, and the stories that each person told allowed the participants to come to know one another. The team contemplated drawing a diagram depicting the canyons of disconnection, but felt that this exercise might result in losing the power of the women's stories if the focus moved to the disconnection.

Insights and Analysis

The research team came to realize that telling the stories was the most powerful action we could take to transform the pattern of racial stereotyping, prejudice, and racism that existed in our community. It was decided that a narrative representation would be best. The team sought the assistance of Nothando Zulu, from the Black Storytellers Alliance. She helped us weave the stories representing the major data themes from the various communities of color into a single narrative. Eight women representing the various aspects of the community performed the narrative before the advisory council as a reflection of the pattern of the community. Then the large group of women was divided into eight smaller groups to reflect and report back to the large group on what data were missing in the narrative and what actions the group wanted to take. The women in the small groups affirmed that the narrative accurately captured their experience and began to develop actions as insights unfolded.

One action taken was the videotaping of the narrative performance to show it to the larger community and the commitment to include women from the various communities of color when presenting the narrative so as to engage the community in dialogue. Another action was the development of monthly "Let's Talk about Race" forums where young women could share personal experiences of racism. These efforts gave individuals the opportunity to get advice from older women on how to deal with racism and to understand that patterns that emerged could point to aspects within the community where systemic change was needed.

The process of community dialogue and action planning is ongoing. The larger community has been involved in a widening circle of dialogue through presentations of the data/narrative performance at community forums, healthcare in-service trainings, and community radio and television. These presentations always invited feedback to expand the dialogue and insights gained.

The dialogue has been rich and insightful, as the researchers seek to understand the complex nature of health and community for multiple groups of women of color affected by racism. As the research process evolves, transformation is occurring as stories are shared. For example, healthcare providers suddenly understand how to improve their care as they listen to African American women speak of going to a healthcare provider and not being touched. In another example, Latina women reported having a fear of deportation every time they went to the emergency department. For their part, Hmong women described their belief that it was better to use traditional medicine or go to a shaman than to the clinic, where they might be hurt or even killed. Through this dialogue, the concept of community and what constitutes appropriate health care is in the process of being reshaped.

The women who were part of this study see health as holistic. Half of the women who listed themselves as *healthy* on the demographic form also reported having at least one significant health problem. Half of the women who stated they were *not healthy* reported having no medical or mental health problems. The women in this community validated Newman's perspective of health as being more than simply the absence of disease. This recognition has implications for the community health center, which currently gets reimbursed for the diagnosis and treatment of physical diseases and problems.

Study Findings

The CCoEWH is in the process of generating new research questions to engage the community. In the initial study, spoken narrative was used to reflect patterns of health back to the community. Future research might consider other methods of engaging a community in pattern recognition, such as diagrammatic representations. Whatever representation strategies are used at a particular point to understand the community, the pattern will continue to change as the health of the community evolves, never staying static but constantly being revised. As the pattern is presented and reflected upon, new insight is gained and transformation ensues, thereby changing the pattern. It is an ongoing cycle of dialogue, reflection, and action. The major findings of this study are being prepared for publication and have also been reported in the master's theses of Amaiwaku-Rushing (2003), Fitzgerald (2003), and Ollom (2003).

Conclusions

When nurses enter into a process of fully open dialectic engagement with communities, the insight takes on added dimensions. The greater the diversity of the participants in the dialogue, the greater the insight potential. It is essential that each dialogue engender mutual respect, honesty, and fully open attentiveness to that which is most meaningful in participants' experiences and relationships. A wider view of the whole is seen when community members with seemingly opposing perspectives are engaged in the dialogue. The researchers in the investigations presented here purposefully sought out "critical friends." From the community issues perspective, the theoretical perspective, and the methodological perspective, "critical friends" can challenge our view and process. Over time, however, when critical friends are engaged in the dialogue, the view of all participants is transformed and the "critical friends" are no longer at the critical edge. Through this process, the circle widens and new voices and perspectives are sought. It is in this tension that the horizon of potential insights and actions becomes broader and clearer. Newman's theory of health as expanding consciousness has profound implications for transforming community health nursing practice.

References

Amaikwu-Rushing, L. (2003). *The experience of women and girls of color in North Minneapolis as it relates to the interplay of health, well-being, and racism.* Unpublished master's thesis, College of St. Catherine, St. Paul, MN.

Connor, M. (1998). Expanding the dialogue on praxis in nursing research and practice. *Nursing Science Quarterly*, 11(2), 51–55.

Endo, E. (1998). Pattern recognition as a nursing intervention with Japanese women with ovarian cancer. *Advances in Nursing Science*, 20(4), 49–61.

Endo, E., Nitta, N., Inayoshi, M., Saito, R., Takemura, K., Minegeshi, H., Kubo, S., & Kondo, M. (2000). Pattern recognition as a caring partnership in families with cancer. *Journal of Advanced Nursing*, 32(3), 603–610.

Fitzgerald, D. (2003). *The experience of adolescent girls of color in North Minneapolis as it relates to the interplay of racism, health, and well being.* Unpublished master's thesis, College of St. Catherine, St. Paul, MN.

Jonsdottir, H. (1998). Life patterns of people with chronic obstructive pulmonary disease: Isolation and being closed in. *Nursing Science Quarterly,* 11(4), 160–166.

Jonsdottir, H., Litchfield, M., & Pharris, M. D. (2003). Partnership in practice. *Research and Theory for Nursing Practice: An International Journal,* 17(1), 1–13.

Kiser-Larson, N. (2002). Life pattern of Native women experiencing breast cancer. *International Journal for Human Caring,* 6(2), 61–68.

Lamendola, F. P. (1998). *Patterns of the caregiving experiences of selected nurses in hospice and HIV/AIDS care.* Unpublished doctoral dissertation, University of Minnesota, Minneapolis, MN.

Litchfield, M. (1993). *The process of health patterning in families with young children who have been repeatedly hospitalized.* Unpublished master's thesis, University of Minnesota, Minneapolis, MN.

Litchfield, M. (1999). Practice wisdom. *Advances in Nursing Science,* 22(2), 62–73.

Moch, S. (1990). Health within the experience of breast cancer. *Journal of Advanced Nursing,* 15, 1426–1435.

Newman, M. A. (1976). Movement tempo and the experience of time. *Nursing Research,* 25, 273–279.

Newman, M. A. (1979). *Theory development in nursing.* Philadelphia, PA: F. A. Davis.

Newman, M. A. (1982). Time as an index of expanding consciousness with age. *Nursing Research,* 32, 290–293.

Newman, M. A. (1986). *Health as expanding consciousness.* St. Louis, MO: Mosby.

Newman, M. A. (1990). Newman's theory of health as praxis. *Nursing Science Quarterly,* 3(1), 37–41.

Newman, M. A. (1992). Prevailing paradigms in nursing. *Nursing Outlook,* 40(1), 10–13.

Newman, M. A. (1994a). *Health as expanding consciousness* (2nd ed). New York, NY: National League for Nursing.

Newman, M. A. (1994b). Theory for nursing practice. *Nursing Science Quarterly,* 7(4), 153–157.

Newman, M. A. (2002). The pattern that connects. *Advances in Nursing Science,* 24(3), 1–7.

Okhlke, S. M. (2002). *The lived experience of adolescents with type 1 diabetes and their transition to autonomous diabetic care.* Unpublished master's thesis, College of St. Catherine, St. Paul, MN.

Ollom, K. (2003). *The experience of women and girls of color in North Minneapolis as it relates to the interplay of health, well being, and racism.* Unpublished master's thesis, College of St. Catherine, St. Paul, MN.

Pharris, M. D. (2002). Coming to know ourselves as community through a nursing partnership with adolescents convicted of murder. *Advances in Nursing Science,* 24(3), 21–42.

Picard, C. (2000). Pattern of expanding consciousness in midlife women: Creative movement and the narrative as modes of expression. *Nursing Science Quarterly,* 13(2), 150–157.

Tommet, P. (2003). Nurse–parent dialogue: Illuminating the pattern of families with children who are medically fragile. *Nursing Science Quarterly,* 16(3), 239–246.

CHAPTER NINE

CREATING BALANCE: RHYTHMS AND PATTERNS IN PEOPLE WITH DEMENTIA LIVING IN A NURSING HOME

SUSAN RUKA

Introduction

Living with the diagnosis and gradual, progressive decline associated with dementia requires courage, understanding, and strength for all who are touched by the illness. The journey of the illness is chaotic, devastating, and frightening for the person with dementia and the grief-stricken family. People with dementia suffer many losses throughout the illness experience but they never lose the ability to feel emotions (Mahoney, Volicer & Hurley, 2000; Raia, & Koenig-Coste, 1999). The behavior of this population is a language, primarily used to communicate emotions, concerns, and desires, but it is not well understood by others. There is a pressing need to create care environments that emphasize an understanding of behavior so as to maximize quality of life for this large, growing, and vulnerable population.

More than 1.56 million people live in nursing homes in the United States, and the average length of stay in such a facility for a person with a chronic illness such as dementia is 2.9 years (Maas & Specht, 1999). For many of the United States' elderly, the nursing home is not just a place where people receive care—it is their home and their way of life. To many people, home is a restful, congenial, and comfortable place where they can find solace and replenish their spirits. The same cannot be said for many of the elderly living in nursing homes. The nursing home routines, programs, and activities; the residents and staff; and the social and physical milieu—all have major impacts on the quality of life of residents. The inability of the person with dementia to verbally communicate information, desires, and preferences does not change that individual's needs. Nursing home residents, particularly those with dementia, are highly dependent on staff for not only direct care needs but also socialization and opportunities to experience laughter, pleasure, and even joy.

HEC and Creating the Environmental Model of Care

An environment of care that specifically addressed the needs of elderly patients with dementia was purposefully developed at the Merriman House, a 45-bed nursing facility located in north-central New Hampshire. A theoretical foundation, supported by research and driven by a philosophy that reflected a holistic perspective, was the basis for this practice model—namely, Margaret Newman's theory of health as expanding consciousness (HEC). Pattern recognition is a way to come to know person grounded the patient care experience (Newman, 2002). Dementia-related memory loss and the inability to communicate verbally may complicate the caregiver's ability to determine and interpret the meaning underlying the pattern. Based on observed behavioral patterns and information offered by families and friends, pattern recognition can provide caregivers with insight to support the connection between the person with dementia and the caregiver.

The creation of a mutual caring relationship results from the connection between the individual/family and the caregiver. All of the participants benefit from this relationship. The increased understanding and knowledge of the person enhances everyone's quality of life. When the person with dementia is understood and accepted for who he or she is in the moment, a shift occurs in the focus during this final stage of life in the nursing home. The person becomes an active participant in the therapeutic relationship, rather than just a recipient of custodial care. This shift in thinking reflects a philosophy distinguishing this model of care from that employed in traditional nursing home care. The unfolding pattern reflects the experience of the whole. Pattern informs caregivers and supports the person with dementia's transition through a period of uncertainty until a new rhythm is established in the movement toward an expansion of consciousness.

Within this model, caregivers also experience satisfaction and fulfillment resulting from participating in a caring and meaningful relationship. Long-term care nursing—and particularly the care provided in nursing homes—is viewed by the public and much of the nursing community as a passive process consisting of providing custodial care in the final stage of a person's life. For many, this time is not viewed as an opportunity for growth, expansion of consciousness, or formation of dynamic and meaningful relationships. However, when care is viewed though the lens of Newman's theory, the nature of the relationship between nurse, resident, and family changes. The art of nursing is actualized in the opportunities for creativity in nursing practice prompted by the interactions of the patterns of the nurse, resident, and family.

Dementia and the Family

The journey of dementia may be the most difficult for the family. People with dementia may spend most of their time living in the moment, interrupting connections to the past and often to their families. The caregivers form a relationship with the person as he or she is "now," coming to know and appreciate the person for who he or she is today. The family, however, faces the reality of having known the person as the individual was in the past while trying to continue a relationship based on how he or she is now. The family serves as the bridge between the two worlds of the person with dementia. They find comfort in knowing that the care of their loved one is based on knowing and valuing the person both as he or she was and as he or she is now. This sense of comfort may dull—but not eliminate—the pain associated with loss of the person as he or she was in the past. Forming caring and supportive relationships with families is an essential aspect in creating care environments for people with dementia.

The Model

The vision of a therapeutic environment that promotes healing and comfort by valuing the person with dementia guided the evolution of the model of care at the Merriman House. Maximizing strengths, minimizing limitations, and, most importantly, fostering unconditional acceptance of the person with dementia were essential components of the building process. However, while the vision of a therapeutic environment was unwavering, the actual creation and operationalization of the care environment proved far more difficult.

The analogy of an impressionistic painting may be used to illustrate the development of the model. The painting provides the observer with an impression and sense of the scene, but the details are not clear. The same was true in the development of the care environment. As the model evolved, the creators had a sense of what they sought to develop, guided by an image similar to that of an impressionistic painting. The staff at Merriman House knew when something was not right, but we did not always know what to do to make the original image become a reality. This uncertainty frequently resulted in frustration, confusion and disequilibrium. Uncertainty is uncomfortable, and some good staff members, craving stability, left the facility in the early stages of the development of the model of care. Others stayed and joined in the discovery process, trusting that we could reach the image in the painting. The pattern manifested within the framework of Newman's theory reflected periods of chaos followed by periods of enlightenment as the care model moved to an expanded level of consciousness. Dealing with the uncertainty was difficult at times, but the team trusted in the process, and the results were liberating. Eventually, as the process evolved, a critical mass emerged and the image in the picture became a reality.

Promoting Comfort

People with dementia are often in a state of chaos, experiencing emotions without the ability to rationalize the origin or meaning of their emotional turmoil. Chaos may be defined as a time of dramatic change. Naomi Feil (1993), a pioneer in improving the lives of people with dementia, described it as being unable to modulate or regulate one's feelings. These feelings and emotions are released without the social filters utilized in the past, and may be related to a multitude of causes. The causes range from the inability to communicate physical discomfort such as hunger, thirst, pain, or fatigue, to more deeply embedded feelings of loneliness, inadequacy, depression, or fear, which often stem from events occurring earlier in their lives. The person with dementia often appears "stuck" in a painful time of his or her life.

Exemplar

Mary was abandoned by her mother for the first five years of her life and spent the remainder of her childhood with her mother randomly entering and leaving her life. During adulthood, the same pattern involving broken trusts continued along with feeling devalued by her husband. As her dementia advanced, Mary spent much of her time in the nursing home anxiously searching for her mother. The staff attempted to meet her emotional needs and help Mary find peace and comfort. She referred to several of the staff members as "mama" and derived comfort by remaining physically close to those caregivers. Mary accepted and returned hugs and other signs of affection. Before her death, Mary's family was contemplating a move out of state. They made the difficult decision not to have Mary accompany them and move to a different nursing home. The family believed that for the first time Mary felt secure and safe, and they chose not to disrupt the sense of peace and comfort she was experiencing.

Promoting comfort in the person with dementia is a goal in the model of care. Comfort is a substantive need throughout life and, as such, it must be achieved before attention can be directed toward the process of healing, which includes a peaceful death (Malinowski & Stamler, 2002). The word "comfort" is derived from the Latin *confortare*, which means "to strengthen greatly." This definition of comfort is consistent with the theory of HEC. The nurse supports the person with dementia through a period of uncertainty. When a sense of balance is achieved through the promotion of comfort, the person's life may take an unanticipated direction. This new direction is characterized by greater connectedness, freedom, and the formation of caring new relationships, all of which are manifestations of expanding consciousness (Newman, 2002).

Creating a "Comfort Zone"

The care environment focuses on determining a *comfort zone* for each person (Ruka, 2003). That zone represents a balance of emotions and behaviors. Promoting comfort by maximizing positive emotions and behaviors and minimizing negative emotions and behaviors enhances quality of life. Patterns of behavior represent expression and meaning, shaping the quality of life experienced by the person with dementia. Tension exists between supporting those behaviors that allow the person to experience joy and a passion for life and avoiding those behaviors that are distressing and painful. The comfort zone is more than the blunting of distressing behaviors; it is the creation of a balance of behaviors and emotions that is unique to the person and enhances quality of life.

The borders of the comfort zone are flexible and dynamic, influenced by both intrinsic and extrinsic factors. Patterns of specific behaviors interact, resulting in varying degrees of comfort. The rhythm of the individual behaviors and overall pattern is considered in light of what is known about the person's life pattern, style, dreams, desires, and preferences, before the onset of dementia. Thus the comfort zone is unique for each person.

The ability to recognize pattern is instrumental in developing the comfort zone for each person. Key concepts are that wholeness identified in pattern and the behavior is an indicator of pattern (Newman, 1999). Behavioral manifestations help make a pattern recognizable. The explicate pattern of the person with dementia is manifested by behaviors; underlying these expressions is an implicate pattern that is the true person. The caregivers search for meaning in the expressed behavior and seek to understand and connect with the whole person.

Recognizing Pattern and Dementia

The visual image of an ocean scene is used to represent explicate and implicate pattern. The picture of a beach with lapping waves and sandy shores can be used to illustrate the explicate pattern or behavioral pattern of the person. The implicate order or true person is represented by the illustration of life under the sea, complete with swimming fish, whales, coral reefs, and vegetation. If we believed the ocean consisted of just the sandy beach and lapping waves, we would miss the incredible undersea experience. The same is true if the behavioral manifestations are accepted as the only representation of the person with dementia. The caregivers form a bond and assist the person's move to a new order, balance, and comfort.

Exemplar

Jean came to the nursing home following a life filled with conflicted emotions, restlessness, and unease. She had learned to close herself off emotionally with biting sarcasm and by physically moving back and forth across the country. When Jean first came to the nursing home, she exhibited anxiety, discomfort, and restlessness. She continually moved around the facility, unable to relax or be still physically or emotionally. Gradually Jean became quieter and enjoyed spending most of her time around the nurses. She would frequently tell the nurses, "I'm scared," and the staff would provide her with comfort, touch, and reassurance. She had never been able to share any feelings and sentiments with her family because she had distanced herself emotionally. Jean began to laugh and talk with the staff. Later she became more open, and told her daughters, "I love you." Jean and her daughters formed new caring relationships. As one of her daughters described the experience, "I see the potential in her that she was never able to actualize. She has such a big hole inside of her—she is gradually filling it with the love she can now accept. I think she will live a long time because she is finally able to accept and show her love and emotions and it will take time to fill that hole." Throughout Jean's stay in the nursing home, her behaviors changed, suggesting a greater sense of comfort and peacefulness.

The Care Model for a Nursing Home

The leadership philosophy at Merriman House emphasized respect for person, collaboration, and teamwork. Many long-term care facilities have used hierarchal management structures that failed to promote understanding of the person's individuality. This care model expanded leadership and management horizontally rather than vertically. The leaders remained visible and accessible, acting as role models for the facility's philosophy of care.

The staff at Merriman House were mentored and provided with the tools and skills necessary for success in this nontraditional management structure. The leaders were expected to maintain the vision and guide the staff in its fulfillment. Staff were encouraged to become open, peeling away the outer layers of protection and defenses that are commonly used in most work settings. This openness allowed for new patterns of interaction among the staff, residents, and families, resulting in enhanced understanding and connection. This openness among the staff and the associated vulnerability needed to be treated with care and respect by all involved. Those in leadership positions, both formal and informal, had an additional responsibility not to misuse the power associated with their position. Instead, they allowed their influence to guide the group toward an expanding level of consciousness.

The leaders continually worked at trusting in the process to avoid reverting to traditional management styles, which have repeatedly proved to be unsuccessful, particularly in long-term care. This effort was especially difficult in times of uncertainty and chaos; during these times, leaders needed to let the theory be their guide. The leaders themselves needed to see the periods of chaos and disruption as opportunities for movement toward a new awareness and expanded level of consciousness. In turn, they communicated this belief to the remainder of the team.

Nurse case managers (NCMs) coordinated holistic and comprehensive care for the residents. Each NCM helped integrate all the available pieces of information, discovered ways to obtain new insights about the resident, involved and supported the family, and served as an advocate for the person with dementia. Families often confided in the NCMs, sharing concerns and in-depth information about the residents. Staff would bring observations and clinical experiences to them. NCMs then used this information to create a comprehensive picture of each resident and share the information with rest of the staff.

The resource or staff nurses provided daily leadership, direction, and guidance to the direct-care staff. They used clinical skills and knowledge of the person to aid in pattern identification, and to discover and implement the care approaches needed to promote comfort. The resource nurses served as the bridge to practice, linking the direct-care staff and the NCMs. In particular, they acted as role models and formed caring relationships with the residents and their families. Resource nurses were instrumental in implementing the leadership philosophy. However, the challenge remained to find a balance that appreciated the value of each staff member, promoted respect, generated self-esteem, and provided the structure needed to maintain the vision of the model.

The Licensed Nursing Assistants (LNAs) provided the majority of direct care, spending the largest amount of time with the residents. The LNAs were highly involved in identifying the residents' patterns and determining therapeutic approaches. They were encouraged and supported in developing caring relationships with the residents and the families. In general, the LNAs had little education and few opportunities to practice the communication, problem-solving, and team-building skills required for this practice model. Formal systems in the model of care supporting the skill development included peer mentoring, coaching, a recognition program, and ongoing education and staff development. More importantly, the formal programs were supported by the provision of ongoing feedback and communication by the leaders, resource nurses, and peer mentors. This ongoing dialogue encouraged the development of openness and connectedness among the team members. The connectedness and mutuality experienced by team members could then be extended to the manner in which care was provided to the residents and families.

An important goal of the therapeutic activity staff was the maximizing positive emotions and feelings. The activity staff was not generally involved in providing direct care, which by nature emphasized a sense of dependence and vulnerability. Therapeutic activities were directed toward nourishing the person's spirit and supporting worth and value. Activities for persons with dementia were designed to use all five senses to make connections, as well as to prevent boredom and stimulate pleasure and satisfaction.

The interdisciplinary team (IDT) met weekly to discuss concerns regarding resident care, accurately determine needs and goals, and make recommendations for changes in the plan of care. The team consisted of the NCMs, administrator, director of nursing, resource nurses, LNAs, registered dietitian, activities coordinator, and the residents' family members if possible. Each resident's assessment data and plan of care were reviewed on a quarterly basis. Family members were invited to attend the meeting when this care plan was discussed.

Each week the IDT members had the opportunity to discuss additional issues regarding residents who might not be due for a routine review. General categories of concern, including behavioral issues, were also reviewed each week. Team members brought forward resident issues, requested input from the team, validated concerns, obtained suggestions for care plan recommendations, and assigned responsibilities for interventions.

Each care element was planned to move toward the goal of complementary healing, identifying pattern and coming to know the person, and creating an environment of care that fostered relationships. The IDT provided opportunities for the team members to become aware of their own patterns as well. This awareness enhanced the team's ability to connect with and understand the residents. Personal awareness and insight also fostered better relationships among team members. The caregivers became more attuned to the implications of the interaction among individual patterns, thereby improving the team's ability to provide quality care.

Rhythm of Care: Synchrony

Caregivers need to understand the rhythm and pattern to become synchronous with the person. Moving in synchrony fosters caring relationships and brings with it a sense of closeness and unity. Caregivers identify the value of moving in harmony with the person with dementia, but they also identify the difficulty in developing a synchronous relationship. It is much easier to develop a synchronous relationship when the rhythm of a pattern is recognizable, clear, and predictable. It is more challenging to synchronize with another person when his or her pattern is irregular, indefinite, or arrhythmic (Newman, 1999).

People with dementia characteristically exhibit variability in their behaviors, emotions, and pattern (Algace et al., 1996; Bourgeois et al., 1996; Mahoney,

Volicer & Hurley, 2000). Although this variability may appear chaotic, it is a form of expression indicative of the rhythm and interaction of the person with his or her environment. Identifying the pattern and forming the relationships, however, is merely the beginning of assisting the person with dementia to an expanded level of consciousness. Newman wrote of the need for the nurse to enter into a partnership with the client and "dance their dance" (1999, p. 229). Of course, dancing is associated with a sense of harmony, as the two partners move together, form a connection and create a partnership in the moment.

Caregivers need to not only dance the dance, but also allow the person with dementia to take the lead. In their desire to help, caregivers may attempt to take the lead in making decisions about what is best for a vulnerable person. Patience is needed to pause and wait, allowing people with dementia to behaviorally express themselves. Promoting comfort begins with the search for the meaning underlying the behavior. Caregivers should develop an understanding of why the person is using a particular behavior and then evaluate the need for intervention. When the behavior reflects a person's inability to meet a need on his or her own, it is appropriate to intervene. The person may be hungry or thirsty or in physical pain and is dependent on the caregiver to alleviate the discomfort. At the same time, the person may have a need to release an emotion such as grief or frustration and should be allowed to express it behaviorally. Forming a synchronous relationship with the person provides the caregiver with insight into interpreting the meaning of the behaviors.

Exemplar

Patricia spent much of her time frenetically pacing the halls of the facility, making continuous repetitive verbalizations. She walked staring straight ahead and without making eye contact with staff, frequently stopping to feel objects on the walls. Patricia's husband wrote a short story referencing some of the meaningful events in her life. The story, complete with photographs, was posted in the hallway of the facility. The stories described a vibrant, bright, and warm woman with a zest for life. Patricia's professional identity was a strong component of her personality. She had a doctorate in public health and was a dynamic and engaging teacher who was popular with her students.

The staff began discussing Patricia's life story with one another. As the staff became more familiar with her story, their relationships with her changed and it became easier to interpret her rhythm and pattern. Patricia began to spend more time in the office resting in a rocking chair. Because of her past, the office was a more comfortable and familiar place for her. Patricia grew increasingly relaxed and began making eye contact with staff. Often, she would pause as she walked about the unit to smile and reach out to staff. Patricia seemed to find comfort in the knowledge that the caregivers now knew her story. Discovering synchrony and learning to "dance her dance" resulted in a greater sense of peace and understanding for all involved. Learning the individualized behavioral language used by each person involves paying attention to the subtleties, as well as being open and receptive.

A Work in Progress

The care environment remains a work in progress. The staff continues to add color and brush strokes to the impressionistic painting that is Merriman House's model of care. The development of this model is dynamic and continues to evolve and move in new directions. Although periods of uncertainty and transition continue to occur, the staff is more comfortable and trusts the process of allowing a natural unfolding of the pattern of the care environment. Continued evaluation of the effectiveness of the model for the residents and their families will provide more evidence about the links between Newman's theory of HEC and its impact on care. When pattern analysis is used to examine behavior, patients and staff change and relationships are transformed. Developing ways to know the patient's experiences can also help guide the future and inform the present by reflecting on the past (Ruka, 2003).

References

Algace, D., Beck, C., Kolanowski, A., Whall, A., Berent, S., Richards, K., et al. (1996). Need-driven dementia-compromised behavior: An alternative view of disruptive behavior. *American Journal of Alzheimer's Disease, 6,* 10–19.

Bourgeois, M., Burgio, L., Schultz, R., Beach, S., & Palmer, B. (1996). Modifying repetitive verbalizations of community-dwelling patients with AD. *The Gerontologist, 37*(1), 30–39.

Feil, N. (1993). *The validation breakthrough: Simple techniques for communicating with people with Alzheimer's-type dementia.* Baltimore, MD: Health Professionals.

Maas, M., & Specht, J. (1999). Quality outcomes and contextual variables in nursing homes. In: A. S. Hinshaw, S. L. Feetham, & J. B. Shaver (Eds.), *Handbook of clinical nursing research* (pp. 655–663). Thousand Oaks, CA: Sage.

Mahoney, E. K., Volicer, L., & Hurley, A. C. (2000). *Management of challenging behaviors in dementia.* Baltimore, MD: Health Professionals.

Malinowski, A., & Stamler, L. L. (2002). Comfort: Exploration of the concept in nursing. *Journal of Advanced Nursing, 39,* 599–606.

Newman, M. A. (1999). The rhythm of relating in a paradigm of wholeness. *Image: Journal of Nursing Scholarship, 31*(3), 227–229.

Newman, M. A. (2002). Caring in the human health experience. *International Journal of Human Caring, 6*(2), 8–11.

Raia, P., & Koenig-Coste, J. (1997). Habilitation therapy: Realigning the planets. *Alzheimer's Association of Eastern Massachusetts,* 3–12.

Ruka, S. (2003). *Effects of reminiscence in promoting a comfort zone: A single subject study of people with dementia in a nursing home.* Dissertation, Boston College, Chestnut Hill, MA.

CHAPTER TEN

CREATING AN ENVIRONMENT OF CARE IN CLINICAL PRACTICE: ADMINISTRATIVE AND PRACTICE PERSPECTIVES

AMANDA COAKLEY

EDWARD COAKLEY

Introduction

It is important that nursing practice be guided by a theoretical perspective and informed by research for knowledge in practice settings to be visible. An organizational infrastructure that fosters professional practice and promotes a climate for scholarship and innovative practice is essential to advance professional nursing. Nursing administrators are in a key position to foster knowledge-based practice to influence cost-effective, quality patient care and improved nurse/patient/family satisfaction. This chapter presents strategies implemented by nurse administrators and clinicians at a major medical center to integrate the theoretical perspective of Newman's (1994) health as expanding consciousness (HEC) and change clinical practice for both the nurse and the patient.

Care Environments and Nursing Administration

Today's U.S. healthcare systems are fast-paced, overcrowded and often technologically driven. The nurse administrator working within this environment seeks to balance workplace demands with initiatives that optimize care and promote professional practice among staff. However, in the current environment of care, administrators spend much of their time projecting future practice needs, designing new organizational structures, and ensuring that resources are available to respond to the demands of a problem-oriented, task-driven patient care environment. For nurse executives who work in large medical centers, much of the daily agenda involves designing and implementing patient and staff data collection systems along with developing innovative processes to support the delivery of patient care. To respond to these demands, administrators analyze data to better determine staffing patterns, identify patient acuity indicators, and budget to accomodate variances. Results obtained from these analyses are used to guide performance improvement initiatives and to assure the delivery of quality cost effective patient care.

The current medical center environment is acute illness oriented and curative driven. Encounters with patients are limited by time constraints and often center on physiologic stability, monitoring disease, and maintaining progress toward recovery, with rapid discharge and some patient teaching to enable patients to recover at home. Nurse administrators participate in organizational strategic planning to address these challenges while identifying and supporting professional contributions to achieve patient as well as organizational goals. The nurse administrator responds by developing strategies to increase capacity (e.g., opening new units to receive more patients), reducing costs (e.g., introducing new technologies to cure pathological conditions), improving patient and employee safety (e.g., with the latest bioprotective devices), and undertaking a myriad of other task-driven and future-focused assignments.

Over the past decade and a half, increased attention has been given to the study of nursing work in an effort to reengineer the healthcare delivery system. Recently, this issue has begun to resurface in a trend that could be termed "reengineering revisited." While the nurse administrator explores new responses to challenging problems, nursing knowledge developments can be used to help inform decisions and redesign care environments so as to optimize outcomes. Such thinking is supported by the American Association of Nurse Executives (AONE) research agenda, which includes work environment and retention considerations (Ritter-Teitel, 2003).

Strategies such as new care models require "out of the box" thinking and new knowledge from a disciplinary perspective to inform their development, such as the case management model developed by Newman, Lamb, and Michaels (1991). A skills/task-based redesign does not permit professional nursing to actualize its potential. As Fitzmaurice and her colleagues (1995) have noted, skill-based contributions, although necessary, do not address the full potential or essential unique worth of nursing. Instead, these contributions often serve to reinforce task-oriented competencies, which fail to reflect the influence of nursing knowledge on clinical judgments and process. Nurses place the future of the profession in peril by failing to identify and practice from knowledge within the discipline. As Mitchell stated, "Health care professionals who define themselves according to a list of tasks and procedures might prepare themselves for replacement" (1997, p. 71). For nurse administrators to optimize the contributions of nursing and improve practice outcomes, they must value nursing science and recognize the influence of nursing knowledge on the nurse–patient relationship and on patient–nurse satisfaction (Spence Laschinger, Finegan & Shamian, 2001).

Nursing Administrators and Nursing Theory

Theory comprises a coherent system of rules and principles, more or less verified or established to help explain or account for known facts or phenomena. "[It] is the unique theories and perspectives used by a discipline that distinguish it from other disciplines" (McEwen & Willis, 2002, p. 25). Nursing theory can be a valuable resource for the nurse administrator, as theory represents logical and intelligible patterns for observations within nursing (Timpson, 1996). It can also be a valuable resource to support reflection and promote clinical innovations. Knowledge embedded in theory can help guide nursing practice and improve patient care. The administrator can use a variety of theoretical perspectives to plan and implement care and change practice settings proactively. When nurses practice purposefully and systematically, they increase efficiency, have better control over outcomes, and are better able to communicate with others (Raudonis & Acton 1997). Newman's theoretical perspective of HEC (1994) can provide a framework for the nurse administrator who wishes to affirm the presence of caring within curative- and market-oriented healthcare systems.

Challenges for Nurse Administrators to Advance Practice

Core curriculum requirements in nursing administration graduate programs are inconsistent (Frank, Aroian & Tashea, 2003), and some programs may omit nursing theory altogether. Also, the trend toward placing a higher value on the master's degree in business administration may further limit familiarity with theory and knowledge within the discipline. While nurse administrators recognize the value of a whole-person approach to care, such as used in HEC-based care, its realization in practice remains a great challenge in an illness-oriented, market-driven, corporate climate. A prevailing perception is that time is precious and that reflection and theoretical thinking are for academics and those who have extra time on their hands. Historically, nursing theory has had a reputation for abstraction and even irrelevance in the minds of many nurses (Timpson, 1996). While some nurse administrators embrace nursing theory (Mitchell, 1997) as a vehicle to guide and inform practice and to generate clinical research, others believe nursing theory has no place in nurse administration. If greater use of nursing theory is to become a trend, it will require an approach that is both clinically relevant and responsive to a dynamic environment of care.

Articulating the content of nursing science and integrating nursing science into practice represents one of the biggest challenges for today's nursing administrators. In the American Nurses Association document *Nursing Administration: Scope and Standards of Practice*, the research standard states that the nurse administrator "creates the environment and advocates for resources supportive of nursing research/scholarly inquiry" (2003, p. 29). This expectation can be realized by the administrator who values and supports necessary for theory-driven nursing practice.

Creating Practice Models

Any effort to create innovative practice models is best anchored in theory. McEwen and Willis (2002) suggest that conceptual models and theories can help guide ways for nurses to communicate their professional values and beliefs and offer a moral/ethical guide to actions. Models and theories can also foster a way to think about practice. Theory-guided practice models have the potential to lead to more coordinated care (Chinn & Kramer, 1999). Models can be thought of as heuristic devices, which help actualize an individual's conceptualization of the world. A nursing practice model is a simple representation that describes the relationship of concepts and ideas about the patient experience. Table 10.1 provides operational definitions of the terminology used when discussing such models.

A professional practice model such as the one developed at Massachusetts General Hospital, Boston, MA, provides scholarly opportunities to advance science and gives direction for examining clinician impact on patient outcomes. This model can be used by nurse administrators to create an infrastructure that supports professional practice and includes elements such as collaborative governance, research, theory, and decision making (Ives-Erickson, Hamilton, Ditomassi & Jones, 2003). Patient-focused care is also informed by professional standards, credentialing and privileging principles, reimbursement practices, and regulatory structures. They can be linked to practice models that reflect the values assigned to the dynamic and therapeutic interaction that occurs between the professional providers and the patient, family, and community regarding issues of health and illness. In this model, the goal of patient-focused care is to ensure that safe, always-improving, and culturally competent patient care is provided to all patients during every encounter. This model provides a framework for

Table 10.1. TERMS RELATED TO MODEL DEVELOPMENT

Model Building: A model is a way of looking at a phenomenon to uncover meaning, pattern, and relationships. It can be imagined as a hologram, which allows the nurse administrator to reflect on complex real-world problems from a "near-far" perspective. Models are approximations of reality and can become a strategy for the nurse administrator to integrate nursing theory and practice into organizational structures and processes. (McEwen & Willis, 2002).

Conceptual Model: Nursing theories share a common meta-paradigm (i.e., nurse, person, health, and environment (Fawcett & Malinski, 1996). These concepts are the foundation of nursing theory and provide a frame of reference for the delivery of nursing care. Nursing models facilitate communication among nurses and provide systematic approaches to nursing practice, education, administration, and research. Conceptual models specify for nurses and society the mission and boundaries of the profession. They clarify the reality of nursing responsibility and accountability, and they allow the practitioner and/or the profession to document services and outcomes.

Professional Practice Model: A professional practice model may provide a means to achieve positive staff perceptions of autonomy and control while managing the realities of changing organizational structures (Spence Laschinger, Finegan & Shamian, 2001). Organizational structures and processes that support professional practice have been linked to positive outcomes for both nurses and patients (Aiken, 2002).

Practice Model: A practice model is a simple representation that describes the dimensions of a nurse's relationship with his or her patient. It can be used to guide the development of focused strategies for delivering nursing care. Practice models are often designed and assessed in terms of patient outcomes, costs, and effectiveness for the healthcare system within which the model exists. The institution's philosophy, staffing patterns, patient population, reporting and documenting mechanisms, reimbursement methods, and communications systems determine which practice model is used.

nurses within the system to explore innovative ways to enhance the care environment, including a HEC-based approach.

Developing Theory-Based Practice: An Exemplar

In an effort to increase discussion around the contributions of nursing knowledge at the medical center, a working group of nurses was designed to examine theory-based nursing practice. Goals were to create a climate that encouraged theoretical thinking within clinical practice settings, and to provide nurses with space and time to engage in dialogue with one another as well as nursing leaders. Other goals included clarifying linkages between theory and practice, creating shared understandings that reflect patient experiences, and articulating more clearly nursing contributions to patient care that are guided by theory-based practice.

During the fall of 1995, a "think tank" was established within the hospital environment to achieve these goals. Initially, the group consisted of a professor/nurse scientist, a nursing administrator, and several nursing leadership support staff. As other nurses learned about the meetings, additional participants from nursing leadership joined the group. Later, many doctoral students from a local university, professors, staff nurses, and members of nursing leadership teams inside as well as outside of the hospital began to attend. The dynamic interaction of nurses from a variety of clinical and academic perspectives enhanced the exploration and achievement of the group's goals. This synergy of theory and practice, which Newman in Chapter 1 and Litchfield in Chapter 7 refer to as "praxis" was realized by all who participated. A conceptualization of a hologram was used to promote a discussion pattern and to illustrate how humans interact with the environment. The holographic model depicts the interaction of persons as an interference pattern of waves emanating from the patterned energy field of each person, becoming the pattern of the whole of the two fields (Newman, 1994). Figure 6.2 presents a visual representation of this model.

Emerging Consensus: The Newman Group

The "think tank" initially included nurses at the medical center enrolled in a doctoral program who had studied the work of Margaret Newman's theory in great depth and felt the theory related to their own philosophy of nursing. The desire to learn more about the theory and its application to practice drew people of like minds together to engage in dialogue and explore possibilities for applying the theory to practice. As the group continued to focus on HEC, the "think tank" grew as other leaders and staff joined the group. The group eventually became known as the "Newman Group."

Group discussions focused on the theoretical components of HEC and this theory's relationship to the work of Rogers (1970). Basic assumptions integral to Newman's theoretical perspective were explored and related to clinical exemplars from practice:

- Health encompasses conditions known as disease.
- Disease can be considered a manifestation of the underlying pattern of the person.
- The pattern of the person that manifests itself as disease is primary and exists prior to structural or functional changes.
- Health is the expansion of consciousness. (Newman, 1997, p. 22)

Group Activities: Reshaping Practice

Members of the group were invited to describe what and how theoretical knowledge guided their current nursing practice. For some group participants, theory had been content studied in the classroom but rarely integrated into clinical practice. The dialogue about the theoretical knowledge within HEC provided an awakening for many participants, who were both intrigued and excited to think about health and illness in a very different way. Many group members began to use pattern recognition (Newman, 1994) as a framework to uncover and reflect pattern. Participants obtained this information by conducting interviews and asking patients to discuss meaningful persons and events that affected their lives. They transcribed the dialogue, developed narratives, and created visual depictions of patterns to reflect the content within the dialogue.

During the group meetings, participants discussed the new strategies they had put in place to consciously "be with" patients and allow time for their stories to unfold. Many clinicians were surprised by the information obtained through asking patients the single question of what was most meaningful to them. As nurses worked with pattern reflection over time (Newman, 1994), they began to appreciate the role the person's story played in informing the current pattern manifestation. "Each pattern is time specific and contains information which is enfolded from the past and which will enfold in the future" (Newman, 1994, p. 72).

Many of the narratives discussed by staff nurses and others were gleaned anonymously from the patient population hospitalized for long-term, chronic health problems. Using HEC-based dialogue gave patients had an opportunity to discuss their unique stories and help the nurse understand their behaviors and expressions observed during their hospitalization. Nurses frequently heard stories that the patients "had never discussed with anyone before." One nurse working on a transplant unit was surprised by the depth of information she obtained from patients in her unit. She noted that, even though many of the patients interviewed had been in the unit for long periods, their stories had remained untold. Using HEC as a framework for assessment, the nurse was able to recognize patterns with the patients and collaborate with them to implement new strategies that promoted choice, comfort, and stress relief. As a whole, the group participants became increasingly aware of how Newman's theoretical perspective guided these encounters and made increasingly visible the importance of the nurse–patient relationship.

Personal and Professional Development Emerging from Group Dialogue

Newman Group members experienced HEC in many ways. Nurses recognized the value of dialogue as a vehicle for professional nurses to connect theory to practice, a perspective that proved transforming for both the nurses and their patients. Group members were able to discuss struggles related to their personal values and beliefs about nursing and the conflicts they experienced when trying to practice professional nursing within a healthcare system that promoted multitasking and technologically oriented care.

The dialogue among the group members revealed that nurses in practice often considered patient disclosure as something to be "checked off" rather than comprehensively evaluated within the context of the individual's story. The group was challenged to develop strategies that led to the creation of a practice environment that optimized theory-guided encounters with each patient.

Meeting as a group promoted learning and became an opportunity for members to grow personally and professionally by expanding their thinking about person, health, environment, and nursing within the context of nursing theory. It was interesting to note that many group participants not initially enrolled in graduate programs went on to pursue higher education, particularly at the doctoral level, and sought to integrate Newman's work into research activities.

Practice Innovations and HEC

Members of the Newman Group incorporated HEC into their own work in different ways. One member of the group explored and developed a theory on reflective practice from a nursing administration perspective and is working on a model to implement this theory in practice. Personal views on unitary humans and Newman's theoretical perspective also provided a framework with which to think about the people and events that shape the role of nursing administrator. An additional insight gained by this administrator in the group was to incorporate reflection as a daily part of the work day. Administrators, nurse managers, and all nursing leaders needed to allow themselves ample time and opportunities to think. While this strategy may not be visible or valued within some current healthcare system structures, it is an important process to enable leaders to stay focused and in the present to listen and engage in dialogue with staff nurses, managers, and others who come to them for advice and direction.

Another group member explored the relationship between patient and provider and energy expenditure during therapeutic touch, a practice identified as part of nursing practice at the hospital (Coakley, 2001). This study was grounded in the Rogerian framework and HEC with the belief that during therapeutic touch, both the provider's and the recipient's pattern "are moving and changing in relation to each other" (Newman, 1994, p. 72). Study results indicated that both partners—nurse and recipient—reported feeling focused and relaxed, yet more energized after the treatment.

A project involving the use of pets in the hospital environment is currently being implemented and evaluated. The presence of pets gives patients an opportunity to stop, connect, and reflect and has served as a catalyst for dialogue. With this intervention, a patient has the chance to connect both with the animal and the staff and to focus on meaning and relationship as a way to optimize health. The presence of pets and the subsequent dialogue are experienced by patients as a way to both get and receive care. This person-oriented health paradigm places dialogue, personal meaning, and quality of life at the forefront and requires a practice mode of collaboration and mutuality (Newman, 1994).

Other participants of the Newman Group have implemented HEC in academic and clinical settings as well as in research investigations. Many of these participants from the original group are reporting their work in this book (A.M. Barron, A. Coakley, E. Coakley, J. Flanagan, C. Hayes, D. Jones, H. Novel-etsky-Rosenthal, and C. Picard). The group has recently been renamed the Newman Scholars Group and continues to meet at a variety of sites to bring together nurses interested in advancing professional development through nursing science and Newman's HEC theory.

Moving Forward: Barriers to Implementation

As participants in the Newman Scholars Group continued their dialogue about HEC and theory-based practice, the administrative members of the group guided their discussion toward the identification of strategies to introduce Newman's theory into practice more broadly. While many staff nurses and advanced-practice nurses found HEC theory interesting and could relate to it on philosophical and personal levels, many struggled with how they would be able to incorporate the model of practice when the healthcare team was focused on the hemodynamic stability and physical needs of the patients. For some, a model such as HEC was seen as setting specific. For example, the nurses believed that the critical care environment did not lend itself to the operationalization of Newman's model, whereas the preadmission clinic was viewed as a "perfect location" for implementation of a HEC-based model of care.

This thinking was grounded in the nurses' belief that for the requisite dialogue to occur, patients must be fully engaged and able to communicate verbally. In settings where nurses were able to talk to patients during the interview and assessment period, Newman's framework could help identify issues and concerns that affect health. The "right" location to incorporate Newman's framework was identified as critical to the implementation of this theory-based practice model. HEC-based practice takes time if the nurse is going to allow the patient an opportunity to talk, reflect, and allow pattern to emerge. The challenge is, however, in creating the environment of care to foster dialogue, an essential component of nursing practice.

Many discussions focused on the importance of using theory to guide professional practice irrespective of the setting, and the value expressed was the need to give patients and families time to be known as persons and to understand the meaning of the hospitalization experience and its context in the life of the patient and his or her family. Nurses understood that anxiety often ran high in both patients and their families. Without adequate time being devoted to dialogue, important information might remain unknown and comfort be compromised. Given that the partnership between the nurse and the patient (and family and community) is the essence of nursing and can be forged in all settings, the barrier to the model's implementation was viewed more as a value issue and needed to be viewed by administration as an expectation of practice.

Summary

Implementing theory-based practice within a fast-paced clinical environment is challenging but possible. It requires valuing, leadership, and commitment by nurse leaders to the contributions that nursing knowledge can make to quality patient care. It also entails recognition that hospitalization has meaning for the person and can be an opportunity for change and growth for both the nurse and the patient (and family). Newman's HEC theory (1994) has implications for both nursing administration and clinical practice. It also provides a framework for the nurse administrator who wishes to affirm the reality of caring within today's largely curative- and market-oriented healthcare systems and structures. The challenge is to sustain practice changes. The long-term effects of creating such a practice environment of care have multiple implications optimizing the practice environment for patients and nurses alike.

References

Aiken, L. (2002). Hospital staffing, organization and quality of care: Cross-national findings. *Nursing Outlook, 50*(5), 187, 194.

American Nurses Association (2003). *Nursing administration: Scope and standards of practice.* Washington, DC: American Nurses Association.

Chinn, P. L., & Kramer, M. K. (1999). *Theory and nursing: Integrated knowledge development* (5th ed.). St. Louis, MO: Mosby.

Coakley, A. (2001) Exploration of energy expenditure between provider and recipient of a therapeutic touch (TT) treatment and the response to (TT) on healthy individuals. *Dissertation Abstracts International* (University Microfilms No. 3021571).

Fawcett, J., & Malinski, V. (1996). On the requirements for a metaparadigm: An invitation to dialogue. *Nursing Science Quarterly, 9*(3), 94–97, 100–101.

Fitzmaurice, J. B., Fernsebner, B., Coakley, E., & Buerhaus, P. (1995). Conceptual mapping of perioperative nursing practice: A validation study. In *Classification of nursing diagnoses: Proceedings of the eleventh conference* (pp. 236–237). Glendale, CA: North American Nursing Diagnosis Association.

Frank, B., Aroian, J., & Tashea, P. (2003). Nursing administration graduate programs: Current status and future directions. *Journal of Nursing Administration*, 33(5), 300–306.

Ives-Erickson, J., Hamilton, G., Ditomassi, M., & Jones, D. (2003). The value of collaborative governance and staff empowerment. *Journal of Nursing Administration*, 33(2), 96–104.

McEwen, M., & Willis, E. M. (2002). *Theoretical basis for nursing* (pp. 27–28, 79–86). Philadelphia, PA: Lippincott Williams and Wilkins.

Mitchell, G. J. (1997). Reengineered healthcare: Why nurses matter. *Nursing Science Quarterly*, 10(2), 70–71.

Newman, M. A. (1994). *Health as expanding consciousness* (2nd ed.). New York, NY: National League for Nursing.

Newman, M. A. (1997). Evolution of the theory of health as expanding consciousness. *Nursing Science Quarterly*, 10(1), 22–25.

Newman, M. A., Lamb, G. S., & Michaels, C. (1991). Nurse case management: The coming together of theory and practice. *Nursing & Healthcare*, 12(8), 404–408.

Raudonis, B. M., & Acton, G. J. (1997). Theory-based nursing practice. *Journal of Advanced Nursing*, 26(1), 138–145.

Ritter-Teitel, J. (2003). Nursing administrative research: The underpinning of decisive leadership. *Journal of Nursing Administration*, 33(5), 257–259.

Rogers, M. (1970). *An introduction to the theoretical basis for nursing*. Philadelphia, PA: F. A. Davis.

Spence Laschinger, H. K., Finegan, J., & Shamian, J. (2001). Promoting nurses' health: Effect of empowerment on job strain and work satisfaction. *Nursing Economics*, 19(2), 42–52.

Timpson, J. (1996). Nursing theory: Everything the artist spits out is art? *Journal of Advanced Nursing*, 23(5), 1030–1036.

PART THREE

RESEARCH AS PRAXIS

CREATIVE MOVEMENT AND REFLECTIVE ART: MODES OF EXPRESSION FOR PARTICIPANT AND RESEARCHER

CAROL PICARD

Introduction

The Newman methodology of research as praxis has been expanded by the author to include additional modes of human expression beyond the dialogue. This chapter addresses the use of creative movement as strategy for participants to express meaning, reflective art as another mode of the researcher's through appreciation of the participant's pattern. These modes of expression are complementary to dialogue, and both may offer participants additional opportunities for pattern recognition and insight.

Relevant HEC Concepts

Consciousness reflects an evolution toward increasing complexity in one's relationship to the world. Self-reflection and pattern recognition are integral to expanding consciousness. Each person's unique pattern is manifested in what is most meaningful to that individual (Newman, 1994). Art and creative movement are modes of inquiry that can illuminate and uncover aspects of self-knowledge, meaning, and understanding.

Newman, Sime, and Corcoran-Perry (1991) identified caring in the human health experience as the focus of the discipline. Caring is nursing's moral imperative, requiring an opening of the heart to what Newman considers the highest form of knowing: "The health perspective demanded by caring is one of unconditional acceptance of the whole. The new rules call for unconditional love which manifests itself in a sensitivity to self, attention to others and creativity" (Newman, 1994, p. 140). As part of HEC theory, nurses are invited to practice with compassionate care, rejecting the values of power and control.

Newman stresses the importance of paying attention to the rhythm of relating or pattern of interacting consciousness (Newman, 1999). This interaction is characterized by flow and movement—that is, a coming together and moving apart—and is best achieved when the rhythms of the persons involved are synchronous. The rhythm of relating to self and others may be enhanced by creative movement, or dance, where the physical act of moving is intended to create meaning.

Creative Movement

According to Laban (1971), movement is the most basic form of self-expression. This conceptualization of a person's inner attitudes affecting quality of movement has been reflective of Laban's holistic view of person. Within this framework, movement serves as the reciprocal link between mental, physical, and spiritual life. Laban found that a richness of movement was a function of the expanding capacity for self-expression. He believed in the potential of movement to foster a broader range of self-expression in people, and he categorized qualities of movement into efforts of time, weight, space, and flow. These qualities he believed to be manifested within a person's movement repertoire and were understood to be a part of a unifying whole. Each person expresses himself or herself in a unique movement effort, reflecting these qualities. Laban's research reflected behaviors and expressions of ethnic groups throughout Europe and the Middle East. Results suggested that a person's movement qualities were connected to the environment and were reflective of the relationship between the person and his or her world. Laban's work complements Newman's HEC theory.

Dance as a Mode of Expression

Dance is a universal mode of expression with capacities for restoration, healing, and heightened self-awareness. From a phenomenologic perspective, coming to understand a person through dance is one path to knowing. Dance has also been a transcendental force used to create altered states of consciousness in religious and healing rituals. It can be a means of movement toward transformation, whereby individuality and common humanity come together (Fraleigh, 1987). When one taps into the deep regions of the dancing body, an opportunity arises to explore those expressions for which there are no words. It is the self-expressive nature of dance that is its most essential feature.

Dance movement therapy literature has contributed a theoretical understanding of the potential power of movement as a mode of self-expression. Research studies have focused primarily on dance and symptom relief for persons with psychiatric disorders (Beaven & Tollinton, 1994; Franks & Frankel, 1991; Lavender, 1992; Milliken, 1990). Nursing research using creative movement has been primarily studied through quantitative modes of analysis with an examination of selected mental health symptoms (Heber, 1993; Goldberg & Fitzpatrick, 1980; Stewart, McMullen & Rubin, 1994). None of the studies that incorporated creative movement into the design employed a hermeneutic approach of reflection on the data generated by creative movement.

As a result of being a modern dancer for 16 years, I had some personal experiences when using movement expressions in class or performances. These experiences led to a deepening of emotional expression and personal insight and prompted me to explore adding creative movement to Newman's research methodology.

Reflective Art

Bauman (1999) invited nurses to examine art as a path of inquiry. Aesthetics is a liminal mode of expression, reflecting meaning and casting light on what has been revealed through artistic expression. Art has a capacity to capture the essence of an experience. When the experience is illuminated, we are caught by it as an arresting awareness of the whole. In that moment, time, space, and boundaries all flow together. Bohm (1998) referred to this confluence as seeing deeply beyond the surface or artifice to the true essence.

Creating artistic expressions is the natural order. Dissanayake (1992), an anthropologist and ethologist, believed that art was a form of embodiment of meaning, making the everyday special, and reinforcing shared significances between people. This author investigated the universality of art-making as a mode of connectedness in cultures throughout the world and believed that postmodern Western people are urgently in need of such ways to communicate with one another. Art as a mode of expression has been valued by many as a therapeutic tool for patients and as a mode of healing (Predeger, 1996; Jonas, 1994; Jonas-Simpson, 1997; Samuels, 1994). Linking art with pattern appraisal could enhance reflection and enhance meaning making.

Cowling (1997) conceptualized nursing praxis from a unitary perspective as pattern appreciation, which is differentiated from pattern analysis. In collaborating with participants to create a profile that included the construction of a story, Cowling used photographs to convey a personal appreciation of the pattern of the whole for the person. As the researcher creates the reflective art as a mode of pattern appreciation, there is an intention to capture the essence of a person's pattern in a new way as it is understood by the researcher (Picard, 2000).

I have used creative movement and reflective art as components of HEC-based studies with mid-life women (Picard, 2000) and with parents of persons with bipolar disorder (see Chapter 12). I have also incorporated reflective art into a study of the experiences of nurses who are cancer survivors (Picard, Agretelis & DeMarco, 2004; DeMarco, Picard & Agretelis, 2004). In addition, I have used creative movement with students (Picard, 2001; Picard, Sickul & Natale, 1998) and artistic reflections in cooperative inquiry exploring the death of a child (Picard, 2002).

Research Design Using Creative Movement and Art

Creative movement and art in research can be examined by considering examples from the study of mid-life women (Picard, 2000). The purpose of this study was to examine the meaning of health for mid-life women by uncovering pattern in narrative dialogue and creative movement modes of expression. Two research questions were addressed:

1. What is the meaning of health as expressed in intentional creative movement and narrative for mid-life women?
2. How is the use of these two modes experienced by mid-life women?

To answer these questions, an in-depth interview was conducted with each of the 17 participants (ages 40–65), followed by a group creative movement experience. The length of the interviews ranged from 50 minutes to 2 hours, or as long as participants needed to speak about meaningful events and people in their lives. The dialogue was followed, within a two-week period, by a creative movement group experience. This group experience lasted 3 hours. Two movement groups were used, one with nine women and one with eight women.

A series of warm-up activities prepared the women to create and perform their own unique movement expression. These activities included trust-building exercises, such as hand-shaking and introducing themselves to the other participants. Then, working in pairs, participants led one another blindfolded around the studio, changing partners until each person had walked with all other participants. The third level of trust building was a trust fall, in which one person stood in the middle of a circle of all other participants and then, with her body held rigid, gave her weight to the group to support. The final exercise was intended to get the group into a reflective mode and comfortable with the studio space. Members were invited to draw their "lifeline" on a large piece of newsprint paper. The participants used this line as a map to move within the studio space, imagining the floor as the paper.

Once the group members were comfortable with one another and with the space itself, each person was asked to reflect on the following question: "If there were a gesture or a movement that could express what is most meaningful for you, what would it look like?" The participants spent time quietly reflecting on this, and creating their solo movements. Then, one by one, each performed a movement, explained what the movement meant to them, and performed it again. Each individual's solo movement was videotaped. The entire group witnessed each performance in silence.

Following the interview and creative movement experience, the researcher examined the audiotapes, videotapes, and transcripts from the dialogue to gain an appreciation of each person's pattern. A piece of reflective art was then generated as a form of pattern appreciation. The process used to create this piece of art included a brief meditation by the researcher during which attention was directed toward a participants' manifested expressions of meaning—in this case, in the interview and creative movement. The symbol that arose during this meditation was then sketched. An artist was enlisted when needed to assist in creating the drawings or in rendering some aspect of the image. For example, a consultation was used to create the figure of a bird in flight. The image was a response to the data, and linked to my immersion in the participants' narratives and creative movements. The artist created the visual to reflect a conceptualization that agreed with my interpretation.

In the second interview, the reflective art and a text-based construing presentation of pattern was shared with each participant, as recommended by Newman (1994). Together the researcher and the participant watched the videotape of the creative movement experience. Each woman was invited to reflect on all aspects of the process. The researcher did not explain the artwork. Instead, this expression was intended to convey to the participant that pattern as grasped by the researcher. As the dialogue continued, participants were free to add, change, or delete parts of the text or the artwork so that it would be as reflective as possible of the emerging pattern.

Findings

Two participants' patterns are presented to illustrate the use of creative movement and reflective art.

Isabel: Creating Balance

Isabel's pattern expression described early experiences of energy bound up in expectations of others and following rules both as a child and in her marriage. This 65-year-old woman identified the most meaningful thing in her life as a search for balance and calm as she began a new transition into retirement. Isabel was one of two children in a family where there had always been a tension between its status as a modest-income family with a minister father and the romantic attitude of her mother. Isabel's mother often denied the reality of her circumstances, instead painting a picture of life different from the one they were actually living. The children in the family did their mother's bidding; otherwise, "She would fall apart. She lived through us and we didn't like it." Isabel was expected to have a career as a writer as designated by her mother. Although she was talented in this respect, it was viewed as a pre-scribed role:

> See, I had a family where we felt pigeon-holed by the parent. They can spot your abilities and label you. I'm the writer but I'm not writing. But that's your role. So you try to find out what it really is. You know, what you really want to do besides what's been proclaimed for you. Why is it that someone can make you feel not good for your whole life?

Isabel married young. Like her mother, she tried to maintain a romantic view of the world. She experienced a period of upheaval when her husband had an affair and left her. For a long time, she felt victimized: "I never saw it coming. Both of us [son and self] were sort of beached by the divorce." Although raising three small children alone was very difficult, she described herself as lucky: "I had a life that I didn't dream of." Despite feeling ill-equipped for single par-enthood and the disruption in her social relationships, this time was period of centering for Isabel: "I wanted something for me. Slowly, with one course at a time. I did it my way." Over the years, she managed to get her master's degree and doctorate in literature, including a fellowship that eased some of the finan-cial burden. Her area of concentration was romantic literature, very much in keeping with her family's pattern. During this period, she developed breast cancer, which was treated successfully and has not recurred.

Isabel's own pattern of seeing a romantic picture of life continued to present problems once she got a college teaching position and sought to move ahead. She lacked publications and was denied promotion. This experience taught her that she needed to prepare for reality differently: "College taught me to hustle." She took a new position and established connections with organizations that could help her better prepare for the promotion process. She also reflected that not noticing the reality of situations had led to being surprised, such as by her husband's affair and daughter's alcoholism and recovery.

Isabel commuted between two residences for many years, from one home near her work to her other, more permanent home near the ocean. As she an-ticipated retirement, she was thinking of how to create a sense of community for herself in the ocean town, something she had in her campus life with col-leagues. She had good but somewhat casual relationships with her seaside neighbors but to live there full-time would require deeper connections. She was also thinking about changing the living space in her home to help her feel a sense of inner calm.

Disease has been a part of Isabel's life off and on. In addition to breast cancer she had been diagnosed with chronic leukemia, but described this illness as being on the "back-burner." It was part of her sense of whole self, but not inhibiting or distressing. Isabel had a good friend who helped her to get through the initial diagnosis, and she reflected on the role stress played in this serious illness experience:

> The balance—the white blood cells are up, the blood pressure, and all that, but you know it's partly an imbalance, maybe in not expressing feelings—or translating them into romantic ways that don't make it okay to feel. [She related a story of not confronting a colleague.] There's a cost, because it builds up and . . . can pop up somewhere else. But when I see it adding into [blood] cells doing the wrong thing—now I'm not 100% sure—it's taken me a long time to see that there could be a lot of different causes.

Isabel was engaged in exploring balance: a pragmatic sense of reality and of hoping for the best outcome. For a good part of her life, she did not feel "in balance" and found that romantic, hopeful perspectives, without more realistic discernment, created problems. These experiences, however, took her to places she never thought possible, such as becoming a professor and chair of a department. She lived out her romantic view of possibilities and hope. Divorce created a pattern of life disruption that shifted her consciousness. She began to identify goals and make choices. A critical point occurred when Isabel was denied the promotion. She began to see life more realistically and was more pragmatic in her decisions. She reestablished relationships with old friends, and enjoyed her professional relationships as well. Isabel's emerging pattern reflected letting go and not caring as much about controlling, outcomes, or what other people were thinking about her actions. Instead, she thought about playfulness, calm, and inner balance, which were reflected in her movements. This pattern was also reflected in her thoughts about leukemia and the balance between red and white blood cells. By connecting with her own inner spirit and with nature, especially the ocean and its tides, Isabel accepted her life as it was and tolerated uncertainty—"the surprises."

Isabel was able to spend more time reflecting and paying attention to her environment, like "the beautiful tree outside my office window." The issue of timelessness was integrated into her talk about retirement. She said, "It's nice to have in life a plateau where you're not being stressed by some emergency." Thanks to this new sense of perspective and an acceptance of her life as lived, she said, "I'm feeling less like I blew it and more that it's worked out for the best. Now I like reality better." During this transition, Isabel was attending more to being than to doing.

Isabel's creative movement was also about balance, stillness, and playfulness. During the movement experience she expressed this by balancing on her right leg, holding her left knee, and raising her right hand in the air. She then switched to the opposite leg, losing her balance and then coming back to center. She opened her arms wide and then began to playfully dance a little jig. Isabel made use of far space in her reaching movements. She stayed on one level and balanced in a narrow plane. Her freewheeling jig ended with a gesture of opening with her arms. She said to the group: "I am working on two things. One is balance. If you lose it, you try again. And the second is getting out of the cage, just wheeling around. Something I don't do much." She said of the creative movement:

> It was very pleasant. You know you get off-balance, then you get on again. That's pretty accurate. I wouldn't have seen it ahead of time, as what I would do. Part of my childhood I didn't mention was falling off a train at 17. I began to see that as a part of the falling down but the getting up again is the thing. You get pretty proud of yourself for being able to balance. And also, if you can't balance . . . that's alright. [She reflected on how she didn't know what she would say to the group about the movement, but as she watched the videotape and saw herself say, "you try again," she commented,] That's when I thought aha! That's true in my family. It's [the movement] not very spiritual. It's more—but it's good enough. It's *my* spirit. The movement part, even though it's hard—it does use *all of you* in the process.

The reflective artwork (Figure 11.1) resonated with her as well:

> Oh yes! It's beautiful. Yeah. Isn't this nice! I like this because that's a real pull. That's such a pull. [She spoke of her exposure to historicism

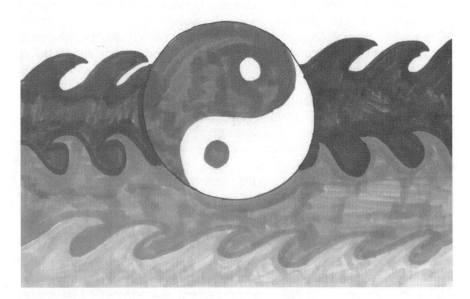

Figure 11.1.   Reflective art for Isabel.

and the shock of realizing multiple ways of organizing reality.] Is this all water, right there? Isn't that wonderful! Cause I am now fascinated when there's tides. I mean I look them up. This is terrific. I just love it. I'll frame it. I'll use it. I'll think about it.

Isabel found the research process a helpful one in gaining some clarity for herself:

Telling, dancing your story seems to be an important thing to do in order to get a sense that there *is* one. It's an artistic process, or a shaping process. And it probably is a shortcutting process, too, in terms of getting insight or getting a sense of self, with a certain immediacy that is at the same time valuable. This is like a fresh way that's effective because nobody but you is really saying/doing whatever it is. You've got a lot of patience and the willingness to listen. So I think it's a shortcut, a valuable way to let people see who they are—to get a fresh look.

Laura: Breaking Down Walls

Laura, age 44, took part in the study at the suggestion of a colleague who encouraged her to call. She did so immediately, "before I lost my nerve." Laura was extremely reluctant to be involved in the movement experience, but stated on the telephone that she needed to take a risk. She described herself as very shy about moving in front of other people with the exception of the children in her classroom.

Laura had spent most of her life, until four years ago, feeling bound to do what others expected of her. There was little feeling of personal choice or freedom. Although she did take some risks as she reflected on her life story, she did not experience those choices that way, internally. Laura protected herself by being overweight. At a young age she felt "different" and was teased by other children. Although she had a supportive family, until recently she had no one else with whom she felt understood. Laura disclosed for the first time, during the second interview, that she had never been asked on a date: "No person on this earth has ever given me a chance, ever in my whole life. I mean, I went on a blind date type of thing but no one ever came up to me and said, 'Wow, I think you are very special. I would like to take you out.'" Friends often looked to Laura for help with tasks or favors. Most of the people in her life were not interested when she wanted to talk about her feelings or what was truly in her heart. These people tended to dwell on their own problems rather than what was good in life and teased Laura if she tried to do otherwise.

A key area of accomplishment for Laura was her talent as a teacher with young children. She was able to recognize when children needed to be known to another. She particularly targeted students experiencing difficulty and sought them out.

Laura's pattern shift occurred when she was 40. During this period, several members of her family became ill. She had a close family and the illnesses served to further open dialogue among them. Laura realized that her goal of being married was not likely to happen, and she decided to change her dream to simply "being happy." During this time, she met a new friend. This was different from other relationships where she was expected to do favors for others:

> That has been the best thing that ever happened to me. We talk about feelings a lot. She is like the first one in my life that knows me—that has taken the time to know me. She's been a wonderful influence on my life and I tell her that all the time. It's so different than before, because she expects me to be nothing but a friend.

Being known was a key ingredient to foster Laura's ability to make choices and not simply follow expectations. This change increased the risk of Laura losing some friends who were not comfortable with her new way of being. But the risk was not a strong enough to diminish this new behavior.

During the group movement experience, Laura was very anxious and shared this fact with the other participants. She was the last participant to do the solo creative movement. It began with Laura slowly walking away from the group. Her head was lowered during this time. She then turned to her audience and began to take progressively larger steps toward them with her hands placed over her heart in a cross-wise fashion. She then made a gesture of peeling off a mask, and knelt down in a prayerful position with her head lowered. Laura shared this response to creative movement and reflective artwork:

> That's me. I removed myself—I kept getting hurt over and over again, and I just couldn't stand it anymore. But my parents never gave up . . . there every step of my life. Then I turned 40 and I was tired of being hurt by everybody, and that's when I stepped back and I removed myself from everyone and everything. I decided I was a good person and I needed to show people that. I hated me and what I stood for, so I started knocking down walls and taking steps, but I'd take two steps forward and one step back. But I kept doing it because of the love of my family. They just kept showing me. They didn't push; they didn't do anything. They were just there. And I took the mask off. I allowed myself to have a lot of masks, and I allowed a lot of people to put those masks on me. Now I'm just me. I'm starting. This is a big step today. I am starting to like me more than I have in my entire life.

During the second interview, Laura responded to reflective artwork (see Figure 11.2) that portrayed a wall with an opening in the center through which a burst of yellow rays of energy is emerging:

> It's very scary—it's who I am, right out there. I like that you've taken the time for this. I mean, I know it's your work, but you've gone deeper than the thesis type of thing. I need this on my wall before I walk out my door every day. This should be framed. I'll just turn this into a pin and I'll just wear it. Or shrink it on the machine [at school] and just put it on. I want that long burst of sunshine.

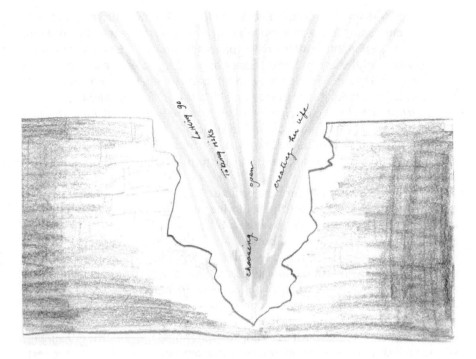

Figure 11.2.   Reflective art for Laura.

Laura also perceived that most of the people in her life did not really know her: "If I gave a blank piece of paper [to them] and said, 'Draw something that symbolizes me,' nobody would even come close to anything like that."

Laura's shift in pattern was manifested by her decision to make new choices, taking risks to connect with new people (i.e., a friend, graduate school), and participating in this research project. She also spoke of learning to break free, such as letting go of her aging sick parents, both of whom have chronic critical illnesses. Laura used a variety of sources and modes of expression to reflect on this journey of self-discovery, including self-help books and journaling. She felt free to share her life at a deep level with certain people. For example, she talked with her parents about their wishes regarding end-of-life decisions and funeral plans, something which she believed would not have been possible a few years earlier.

Discussion

The response of the participants to creative expressions included within Newman's research as praxis process was positive. The creative movement experience provided an opportunity for participants to experience an embodied reflection of the whole in motion. Viewing the videotaped movement provided participants with another opportunity for reflection on the patterning process, as the women saw themselves move in ways that were meaningful to them. Watching the performances of the participants and viewing the tapes, reminded the researcher of the use of sacred dance and other professional interpretive choreography. Through creative movement, participants experienced a heart-felt sense of integration or coherence in their thinking, feeling, and moving.

All except one of the participants asked for copies of the artwork. Through the creative mode of expression and in dialogue, the participants gained a deeper understanding of being known, a key finding in the research overall. The use of reflective art also affirmed pattern and became a resource for further reflection.

The group members' experiences could be likened to old-wisdom traditions of groups such as the Navaho/Dineh, in which a healer thoughtfully reflects on the situation of a person suffering from a problem and creates sand paintings that reflect the pattern of the ill person. Music and dance are also created for restoration (Ramsey, 1991). This research process is one of co-creation, whereby the movement, artwork, and dialogue capture a sense of the whole. Offering all elements contained in the research back to participants for reflection gave them an opportunity to feel truly understood by the researcher, and was a way to rec-ognize their pattern. Some participants were drawn more strongly to one form of expression over another, such as dialogue, performing the creative movement, viewing the creative movement, reviewing the artwork, and examining the text-based construal.

Conclusions

The aesthetic mode of expression is a door to awareness and reflection that opens up possibilities for further investigation. Newman's theory of HEC, along with expanded methodologic strategies, provides a rich opportunity for creative expressions of pattern. Bohm reminds us that "true knowledge and in-telligence does not arise in thought. Rather the deep source of intelligence is the unknown and indefinable totality from which all perception originates" (1998, p. 61). Creative movement invites engagement of the whole person, and the videotape presented offers an opportunity for participants to see them-selves in a different way. Reflective art can express caring presence in a new way.

References

Baumann, S. L. (1999). Art as a path of inquiry. *Nursing Science Quarterly*, 12(2), 111–117.

Beaven, D., & Tollinton, G. (1994). Healing the split: A psychophysical approach to working with sexually abused teenaged girls. *Physiotherapy*, 80(7), 439–442.

Bohm, D. (1998). *On creativity*. New York: Routledge.

Cowling, W. R. (1997). Healing as appreciating wholeness. *Advances in Nursing Science,* 22(3), 16–32.

DeMarco, R., Picard, C., & Agretelis, J. (2004). Nurses' personal experiences of cancer survivorship. *Oncology Nursing Forum*, 31(3), 523–530.

Dissanayake, E. (1992). *What is art for?* Seattle: University of Washington.

Fraleigh, S. (1987). *Dance and the lived body*. Pittsburgh: University of Pittsburgh Press.

Franks, B., & Fraenkel, D. (1991). Fairy tales and dance/movement therapy: Catalysts for change in eating disordered individuals. *Arts-in-Psychotherapy*, 18(4), 311–319.

Goldberg, W. G., & Fitzpatrick, J. J. (1980). Movement therapy with the aged. *Nursing Research*, 29(6), 339–346.

Heber, L. (1993). Dance movement: A therapeutic program with psychiatric clients. *Perspectives in Psychiatric Care*, 29(2), 22–29.

Jonas, C. M. (1994). True presence through music. *Nursing Science Quarterly*, 7(3), 102–103.

Jonas-Simpson, C. M. (1997). The Parse research method through music. *Nursing Science Quarterly*, 10(3), 112–114.

Laban, R. (1971). *The mastery of movement*. Boston: Plays.

Lavender, J. (1992). Winnicott's mindpsyche and its treatment. *American Journal of Dance Therapy*, 14(1), 31–39.

Milliken, R. (1990). Dance/movement therapy with the substance abuser. *Arts-in-Psychotherapy*, 17(4), 309–317.

Newman, M. A. (1994). *Health as expanding consciousness* (2nd ed.) New York: National League for Nursing.

Newman, M. A. (1999). The rhythm of relating in a paradigm of wholeness. *Image: The Journal of Nursing Scholarship*, 31(3), 227–230.

Newman, M. A., Sime, M. A., & Corcoran-Perry, S. A. (1991). The focus of the discipline of nursing. *Advances in Nursing Science*, 14(1), 1–6.

Picard, C. (2000). Uncovering pattern of expanding consciousness in mid-life women: Creative movement and the narrative as modes of expression. *Nursing Science Quarterly*, 13(2), 150–158.

Picard, C. (2001). Expressive techniques: Embodied knowing. In: M. Bradshaw & A. Lowenstein (Eds.), *Fuzard's innovative teaching strategies in nursing* (pp. 149–158). Gaithersburg, MD: Aspen.

Picard, C. (2002). Family reflections on living through sudden death of a child: Cooperative inquiry grounded in Newman's health as expanding consciousness. *Nursing Science Quarterly*, 15(3), 242–250.

Picard, C., Agretelis, J., & DeMarco, R. (2004). Nurses' professional experiences of cancer survivorship. *Oncology Nursing Forum*, 31(3), 537–542.

Picard, C., Sickul, C., & Natale, S. (1998). Healing reflections: The transformative mirror. *International Journal for Human Caring*, 2(3), 29–47.

Predeger, E. (1996). Womanspirit: A journey into healing through art in breast cancer. *Advances in Nursing Science*, 18(3), 48–58.

Ramsey, J. (1991). Poetry and drama in healing: The Iroquoian Condolence Ritual and Navaho Night Chant. *Literature and Medicine*, 8, 78–99.

Samuels, M. (1994). Art as a healing force. In: *Body and soul: Contemporary art and healing*. Lincoln, MA: DeCordova Museum.

Stewart, N. J., McMullen, L. M., & Rubin, L. D. (1994). Movement therapy with depressed inpatients: A randomized multiple single case design. *Archives of Psychiatric Nursing*, 8(1), 22–29.

CHAPTER TWELVE

PARENTS OF PERSONS WITH BIPOLAR DISORDER AND PATTERN RECOGNITION

CAROL PICARD

Introduction

I was introduced to Newman's theory of health as expanding consciousness (HEC) as part of a course experience in the doctoral program in nursing at Boston College. Having been a psychiatric nurse for 30 years, I found that Margaret Newman's work resonated with me quite strongly. The unfolding unidirectional nature of consciousness offered a more accurate way to understand patient experiences than did the traditional crisis theory, where the goal is to return people to their pre-crisis level of functioning. Newman's theoretical position validated for me that the crisis experience was instead life changing and each person seemed to define his or her own path to healing.

This chapter presents research grounded in HEC theory and the experiences of parents of persons diagnosed with bipolar disorder. For many years, I partnered with members of the Alliance for the Mentally Ill, a self-help group for families and friends of persons with mental illness. During this time, I attended the meetings with my undergraduate nursing students. These meetings focused on families offering one another support and information. Students would come to understand the complexity of mental illness within the family through these meetings and related faculty guidance.

While completing my doctoral work, members of the Alliance asked about the nature of my research. I explained my work as a way for individuals to better understand health, and the use of creative movement and reflective artwork to complement the dialogue (Picard, 2000). Members of the group suggested a study with parents of people with mental illness, because "No one has the time to listen to our stories, and we have stories to tell and want professionals to learn about our experience."

The study took place in Massachusetts in partnership with 15 parents of children diagnosed with bipolar disorder. For most of the participants, it marked the first time they were able to relate their personal stories and meanings in as much detail as they desired. The experience of being a parent of a child with mental illness was part of a larger pattern that emerged and reflected the complexity of their relationships as a whole.

Relevant HEC Concepts

An important part of living out HEC as a nurse and researcher is appreciating one's own pattern. Being born into a family with several extended family members experiencing bipolar disorder, I have experienced a limited dose of the energy associated with that illness. As I like to tell my students, I believe that researchers will eventually find that it is possible to get the bipolar trait, like the sickle cell trait, and that trait can serve a person well. I believe I must use this energy wisely and creatively as a way to honor the spirits of my relatives who were challenged by the severity of their illness. This researcher experience is part of my pattern and must be acknowledged as part of the research process.

According to Newman (1994), recognizing pattern takes time spent in reflection and is best supported by dialogue and the presence of another person. Certain events in one's life can be experienced as chaotic or uncertain and are part of the unfolding pattern. When a family has a member who experiences an illness, in this case a mental illness, the disorder can create disruption in the patterns of all members. It is in times of such disruption that nurses often encounter patients and their families. In the HEC model of research, the focus is on an open dialogue, allowing the participants to uncover their patterns by expressing them in their stories. In addition to being present and inviting dialogue, participants in this study had an opportunity to express their patterns in creative movement. The process changed not only the participants, but the researcher as well.

Literature Review

Bipolar disorder is a chronic mental illness and a major mental health problem, with 1–2% of the population being diagnosed in early adulthood. It is typically characterized by a disturbance in mood marked by alternating episodes of mania and depression. The person with bipolar disorder also has disturbances in thought processes, behavior, sleep patterns, and nutrition (Fortinash & Holoday-Worret, 2003). In the prevailing American model of psychiatric care, access to resources for the mentally ill is limited, and family support services are often lacking (U.S. Department of Health and Human Services, 1999).

Rose (1996) recommended that nurse scholars use interpretive research methods to investigate family perceptions of mental illness. A literature review at the time of the study revealed only one researcher who had examined the experiences of families of persons with chronic mental illness guided by Newman's theory and methodology (Yamashita, 1998a, 1998b, 1999). This research was limited to the experiences of families with a member diagnosed with schizophrenia. Given that schizophrenia and bipolar disorder differ in their symptom presentation, the experiences of affected parents may differ as well. Some studies did look at family members where all major mental illness categories were selected for review (Doornbos, 2002; Eakes, 1995; Karp & Tanarugsachok, 2000; Mohr & Regan-Kubinski, 2001; Muhlbauer, 2002; Stern et al., 1999), as well as those studies of parents of persons with schizophrenia (Jungbauer, Wittmund, Dietrich & Angermeyer, 2003; Milliken, 2002). No studies selectively examined the experiences of parents who had children with bipolar disorder. Personal and clinical knowledge of this illness led me to believe that this group of parents might face some unique challenges. A Newman-based model of research was thought to be helpful in uncovering pattern and new knowledge for nursing and other disciplines.

Study Design

A study design based on Newman's research protocol (1994) was developed to incorporate dialogue as well as creative movement as modes of expression for parents of children with bipolar disorders. Findings from a previous study using creative movement indicated that this experience was integrative and assisted in pattern recognition (Picard, 2000). The research praxis is one of engagement in which the consciousness of researcher and participant are shared. Being fully present to participants is essential to the process. Journaling by the researcher was used to reflect on pattern, and a daily meditation practice was kept throughout the research process.

The researcher met with each participant for two interviews/dialogues and one creative movement experience. The procedure was to first interview/dialogue with participants, then a creative movement experience was videotaped in a dance studio, and finally a second interview/dialogue took place. The procedure was completed within a five-week period. The question asked of the participants followed Newman's protocol (1994): "What are the most meaningful people and events in your life?" Each participant was asked a second question prior to the creative movement experience: "If a movement or gesture could capture the essence of that meaning, what would it be?"

Before the second interview, the researcher reflected on the audiotape, transcript, personal experience of the person, and videotape of the creative movement. A text-based diagram was constructed using the person's own words, identifying important events and relationships over time. A piece of reflective art was also created as an expression of pattern appreciation. During the second meeting, the diagram and artwork were shared with each participant. Both the researcher and the participant watched the videotape of the creative movement, and each participant was invited to reflect on his or her story, and the research process.

Findings

Each person's pattern was affected profoundly by his or her child's illness. Several major themes were also observed when looking across participant's patterns, including (1) the lifelong challenge, (2) the need for caring partnerships, (3) the need to regulate energy, (4) uncertainty about the future, and (5) expanding connections. The uncertainty and suffering experienced by the parents were counterbalanced by the possibilities for change and transformation. The demands of their situations did not allow time for self-reflection, and the research process provided that opportunity. The following story describes one parent's pattern.

Ann's Story: A Good Person of Action

Pattern Theme: Lifelong Challenge

Ann was the mother of three boys. Her oldest son Mark, age 16, was diagnosed with bipolar disorder 2½ years ago. Ann was not a stranger to bipolar disorder, as she had a brother with the same diagnosis. In her own family, Ann has always been the responsible one, "the good person of action" to whom others turned in a crisis. She had been very close to her father, whom she still misses every day since his death to cancer. Her mother's long-standing pattern of dealing with problems had been to avoid them. Ann regularly stepped in to fill the gap of parenting with her brother during his illness episodes. Even when Ann's father was very ill, her mother could not acknowledge how sick he was, even in the last week of his life. "She refused to be a part of anyone's care." Ann wished she could count on her mother for support with Mark, but was realistic enough to know that this was not forthcoming.

Until Mark's illness, Ann always believed that "If you behaved, life was a lead-pipe cinch. But it's not true." She believed that because she conducted her life properly, she would be successful as a result, and so would her children. When Marks' illness was manifested as a young teenager, Ann found that it broke through the pretense of assumed goals she had for family: "I didn't even realize I had put those [expectations] on my son."

Ann's life was characterized by many losses, beginning with family stories of losing the family ancestral home in Germany to the Nazis, in addition to the death of her father and the withdrawal of some extended family members since Mark's diagnosis. In her creative movement, Ann shared memories of Mark's peaceful and gentle childhood—"all the tremendously simple, easy things that we take for granted but remember." She had felt so "rooted, secure, down, encompassed: Where did it go?" Ann spoke as she created her movement expression, saying sorrowfully that her son is not the "old Mark" she once knew. This realization was expressed in movement by slowly walking away and looking back, reaching out to her son. Ann wished that her son could grow to do the things he wanted to do. But the feelings of helplessness often overwhelmed her: "My cup of warm milk isn't enough anymore. His world is full of pain I can't touch." In her creative movement, Ann used gestures of shepherding a child, and then losing the connection. The piece of reflective artwork created for Ann was a cup with her words "my cup of warm milk isn't enough anymore" around the edge of the picture.

Pattern Theme: Need for Caring Partnerships

Ann became acutely aware of how much she missed her father at the time of her son's diagnosis. Some family members, friends, and acquaintances distanced themselves as a result of Mark's outbursts and other behaviors. The demands of paying closer attention to Mark and needing to be present at home most of the time reduced Ann's ability to maintain or establish relationships with people beyond the immediate family, which led to a feeling of isolation for Ann. Mark's illness became the focal point for many of the conversations with adults in her life. Ultimately, her lack of satisfying adult relationships caused Ann to realize how important these connections were to her life. Professionals had not been helpful to Ann in her struggle to find a balance between ordinary family life and her son's illness. Their focus on symptom management was a source of frustration:

> We've been sort of under this diagnosis cloud for two and a half years, and we're coming through this fog. Now I think, why not let Mark look at life and just think about other things, you know, not just medication, not just the therapy, not just the psychiatry visits. Last night was our last session with the family therapist, and it was such a relief.

Pattern Theme: Regulating Energy

For almost two years, Ann's energy was bound up in attending to Mark, despite her attempts to balance her energy and the family's energy as a whole. The illness and its related symptoms posed a challenge for everyone concerned. Ann noted that she eventually adapted to Mark's rhythm of energy, as did the rest of the family. "Things may be fine, and then all of a sudden it's too much for him. I have to understand this. The other two boys don't want to be labeled as a sibling of someone with a mental illness. They just want to be themselves." Ann found she had to contain and modulate her personal feelings in ways that could sometimes be exhausting. She maintained a sense of vigilance toward Mark, and she did not realize the trouble he was in until she read his notebooks after his first hospitalization. She worried whether she would be able to trust Mark's behaviors even when he seemed to be doing well.

During this period, Ann had little time for self-care and restoration. Recently, she had become more intentional about carving out some time for herself, without Mark. There had also been little time to tend to her marital relationship. She and her husband loved and supported each other, but most of their conversations revolved around Mark, his schoolwork, and his treatment.

Change: Action, Acceptance, and Letting Go

Ann continued to seek a new form of "normality" in a household that now included a member diagnosed with bipolar disorder. She was letting go of "being perfect, wonderful, and right, and yielded to the goal of redirecting care for myself, my husband, and my children." She was conscious of helping all three boys to "grow to be who they are, and letting Mark be as Mark as possible." This was a newfound ability to accept things as they were and to let go of old expectations. Ann valued the ordinary, such as having dinner together as a family where everyone talked about their day. She took joy in that simple pleasure. This attitude required being focused on the present and letting go of the past as well as future dreams and expectations.

Ann also discovered that Mark's illness created a new role for her among the family and community. This transformation was manifested by a new degree of openness among certain extended family members. Recently, Ann was able to talk with her mother about Mark's illness, something they never did earlier when her brother suffered a similar problem. Now she experienced the beginning of dialogue on a different level. After two years, her mother expressed some sensitivity to the situation and recently attended an Alliance for the Mentally Ill meeting and read materials about bipolar disorder. Ann's brother, who has bipolar disorder, had conversations with Mark that she found comforting. For other extended family members, however, this change has not occurred: "It's hard for them to hear us talk about Mark, because it 'taints' them."

Ann has also reached out to a new church community and received much caring and support. Disclosing and expressing the hardship of living with the illness in her family with church members had "broken down the walls of polite society." Ann now feels that she and her family are truly known and accepted by church members for who they are. She and her husband also began to form an education support group for other family members of children with mental illness. This action was seen as a way to create a sense of community with other parents, and an opportunity to continue to experience mutual supportive connections with others. It was also in keeping with her pattern of doing something "good," even though she has given up the assumption of its protective effect and is accepting of the uncertain elements in her life.

Research Process and Reflection on Pattern

As she used creative movement, Ann had an insight that helped her to express her story. She commented on the value of reflection, movement, and dialogue:

> It just makes more sense. I remember I was trying to tell [my husband] what happened, and I couldn't remember the words, I just remember what the meaning was. But it was very good. It meant a lot to me to do

it. It [the research process] translated the present feelings into actual thinking, instead of just living it.

Reflecting on her pattern of caring for everyone in the family helped Ann clarify the need for personal change. She began to set limits on certain extended family members and was mindful of the energy needed to care for her immediate family. She was also trying to answer an inner "cosmic cry" to visit her father's brother, who lived in another state, before he died. She continued to struggle to regularly find time in her week to reflect on the choices she was making.

Discussion

Having a child with bipolar disorder was experienced by Ann and other participants in this study as a major disruption in their life patterns. Old ways of relating had to change quickly to accommodate the child's new behaviors, energy, and capacity for connection. The chaos within the child's illness pattern was reflected in the participants' own patterns of expression. The complexity of relationships with family and others in the community changed as well. Ann's story was similar to those of other study participants who worked very hard to understand and accept this new element within their life stories. The level of turmoil and distress varied with each study participant and was related to how the illness was expressed by his or her child, self-care resources, and the quality of relationships with family, professionals, and other community members.

The thematic uncovering of "appreciating ordinary moments," such as a family dinner with conversation, was described as a search for normalcy. Participants used this term in two ways: to describe moments of connection and dialogue, and to distinguish them from the feeling of being identified with the disease process. These moments were times of peace in between times of turbulence. This study supports findings by Neill (2002) and Yamashita (1998b) related to the value and pleasure found in the simple ordinary moments and things in life when confronted with highly disruptive moments.

Ann's recent process of letting go of the need to control and accepting her son as he is now indicated an evolution of consciousness similar to findings in an earlier study (Picard, 2000). In that study, letting go was associated with the stage of de-centering in Young's schema of evolution of consciousness (see Chapter 2, Figure 2.1). Ann let go of the illusion of control and perfection, and she began to move toward the process of de-centering, choice, and potential freedom. Ann's experiences with her son's illness enhanced personal awareness, as supported by her husband and church members.

Interactions with mental health professionals were also reflected in Ann's pattern. Although she did receive information about the disease and its symptoms, a lack of caring partnerships with professional staff potentially delayed the process of evolving consciousness and added to the turbulence. With one exception, all of the study participants expressed disappointment or anger with mental health professionals. It is unclear whether these professionals understood how they were perceived by the parents. As a psychiatric nurse this also gave me pause to think: When have I disappointed my patients and their families? Zola (1992) believed that the social construction of illness and society's responses to the person and family can aggravate an already difficult situation. A symptom management orientation with families in need of a caring approach, discounted the full range of their experience and intensified an already challenging situation.

Eakes (1995) found that parents of young people with schizophrenia experienced chronic sorrow about the child's illness. They expressed a need for involvement in the child's care as well as information from mental health providers. Participants in this study spoke of suffering in response to their situation. A Newman-based approach toward care of parents provides a partnership model of care in dialogue that might mediate sorrow and suffering. As Pharris writes in Chapter 8, it is important for the professional community to reflect on its own pattern of interaction with parents, so as to consider how to improve caring partnerships.

Conclusions

Parents of persons with bipolar disorder experience chaos and turbulence as they try to achieve a sense of balance for self and family as a whole. The process of letting go of old expectations and control can help to reduce parental distress and suffering. Nurses and other healthcare professionals can make a difference by creating space and time for partnership and dialogue to support parents in this process. Taking a larger view of the complexity of the family's pattern and being present to parents can support expanding consciousness.

References

Doornbos, M. M. (2002). Family caregivers and the mental health care system: Reality and dreams. *Archives of Psychiatric Nursing*, XVI(1), 39–46.

Eakes, G. G. (1995). Chronic sorrow: The lived experience of parents of chronically mentally ill individuals. *Archives of Psychiatric Nursing*, 10(2), 774–784.

Fortinash, K. M., & Holoday-Worret, P. A. (2003). *Psychiatric mental health nursing* (2nd ed.). St. Louis: Mosby.

Jungbauer, J., Wittmund, B., Dietrich, S., & Angermeyer, M. C. (2003). Subjective burden over 12 months in parents of patients with schizophrenia. *Archives of Psychiatric Nursing*, XVII(3), 126–134.

Karp, D. A., & Tanarugsachok, V. (2000). Mental illness, caregiving and emotion management. *Qualitative Health Research*, 10(1), 6–25.

Milliken, P. J. (2002). Disenfranchised mothers: Caring for an adult child with schizophrenia. *Health Care for Women International*, 22, 149–166.

Mohr, W., & Regan-Kubinski, M. J. (2001). Living with the fallout: Parents' experiences when their child becomes mentally ill. *Archives of Psychiatric Nursing*, XV(2), 69–77.

Muhlbauer, S. (2002). Experience of stigma by families with mentally ill members. *Journal of the American Psychiatric Association*, 8(3), 76–83.

Neill, J. (2002). Transcendence and transformation in the life patterns of women living with rheumatoid arthritis. *Advances in Nursing Science* 24(4), 27–47.

Newman, M. A. (1994). *Health as expanding consciousness* (2nd ed.). New York, NY: National League for Nursing.

Picard, C. (2000) Uncovering pattern of expanding consciousness in mid-life women: Creative movement and the narrative as modes of expression. *Nursing Science Quarterly*, 13(2), 150–158.

Rose, L. E. (1996). Families of psychiatric patients: A critical review and future research directions. *Archives of Psychiatric Nursing*, 10(2), 67–76.

Stern, S., Doolan, M., Staples, E., Szmukler, G. L., & Eisler, I. (1999). Disruption and reconstruction: Narrative insights into the experience of family members caring for a relative diagnosed with serious mental illness. *Family Process*, 38(9), 353–369.

U.S. Department of Health and Human Services (1999). *Mental health: A Report of the Surgeon General*. Rockville, MD: National Institutes of Health.

Yamashita, M. (1998a). Family coping with mental illness: A comparative study. *Journal of Psychiatric and Mental Health Nursing*, 5, 515–523.

Yamashita, M. (1998b). Newman's theory of health as expanding consciousness: Research on family caregiving in mental illness in Japan. *Nursing Science Quarterly*, 11(3), 110–115.

Yamashita, M. (1999). Newman's theory of health applied in family caregiving in Canada. *Nursing Science Quarterly*, 12(1), 73–79.

Zola, I. (1992). The social construct of suffering. In: P. L. Stark & J. P. McGovern (Eds.), *The hidden dimension of illness: Human suffering* (pp. 11–23). New York, NY: National League for Nursing.

CHAPTER THIRTEEN

CREATING ACTION RESEARCH TEAMS: A PRAXIS MODEL OF CARE

EMIKO ENDO

HIDEKO MINEGISHI

SATSUKI KUBO

Introduction

This chapter describes an innovative strategy used to bring a Newman theory-based health as expanding consciousness (HEC) model of care to the clinical setting. Through education and partnership, practicing nurses were able to reflect on their practice and collaborate to create change.

Praxis Model of Care

This praxis model of care is a mutual action research process that involves nurse researchers/educators working in collaboration with practicing nurses. It is grounded in the unitary-transformative paradigm in nursing and bridges nursing research and practice within Newman's HEC theory. The assumptions underlying this praxis model of care include the following:

- Practicing nurses and nurse researchers are open systems. The relation is a partnership.
- Pattern recognition through dialogue facilitates participants' expanding consciousness and includes the transformation of self.
- The unfolding process of nurses' transformation increases practice wisdom and brings changes in nurses' care patterns.

- The process of change is unidirectional and unpredictable. When a change occurs in process, it is transformational.
- Any change emanating from practicing nurses spreads over the whole.

The praxis model of care, as illustrated in Figure 13.1, is an unfolding spiral process; it moves on through integration of the dialogue among the participants at the research/practice project meetings and the nurses' everyday nursing practice. The model being discussed includes eight phases. First, there is a preparation phase, followed by the formation of the project team. The practicing nurses identify a hope they seek to actualize in practice. This hope is transformed into a research/practice proposal, and piloted in practice. The team incorporates a reflective and action process. The proposal is modified as needed and integrated with the reality of practice in a continual process of action and reflection. Lastly, the team presents the project findings. This unfolding process of the praxis model of care is illustrated with a project named "Creating a caring program with patients and their families (clients) in the difficult situation of terminal cancer by applying Newman's theory of health as expanding consciousness (HEC)."

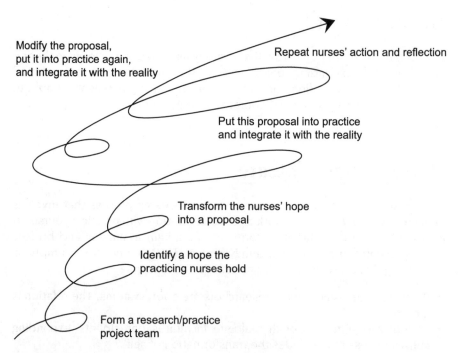

Modify the proposal, put it into practice again, and integrate it with the reality

Repeat nurses' action and reflection

Put this proposal into practice and integrate it with the reality

Transform the nurses' hope into a proposal

Identify a hope the practicing nurses hold

Form a research/practice project team

Figure 13.1. The process underlying the praxis model of care.

Phase 1: Preparing for the Research/Practice Project

This research/practice project was a longitudinal process. The initiators took time to prepare for it, rather than "doing it quickly." All participants needed to know something about Newman's theory. For this reason, the prospective participants, especially the practicing nurses, were provided several opportunities to learn about the theory with the researchers initiating the project. If this was their first exposure to the theory, the nurses would learn about the components of the theory and its application in practice. Because practicing nurses are often strongly influenced by the medical paradigm, the team researchers made an effort to interact with the nurses in practice from the theoretical perspective and created a dialogical environment at study meetings. The theory could then become a part of the process, with transformation occurring in the interpenetration of the initiators' and others' patterns (Newman, 2002).

Each time the research team was asked to come to a unit, it offered the staff nurses an opportunity to learn the theory. Soon the nurses began to understand HEC. Some were attracted to it and could immediately address certain experiences with their clients in the evolving process of consciousness. Although most nurses asked questions about what was correct and what was wrong from the perspective of the theory, the important thing was not to answer them directly but rather to facilitate the emergence of each nurse's own ideas and thoughts. The participants enjoyed the dialogical environment and learning the theory.

Phase 2: Forming a Research/Practice Project Team

At the project initiators' invitation, a research/practice project team formed. The team consisted of a few groups of partnering researchers and practicing nurses. Project meetings were important to inspire creativity, dynamism, meaningfulness, and joy in the unfolding process. Although the meetings included primarily the members of the research/practice project team, they were open so that any practicing nurse could participate. Openness of meetings and communication was critical to provide both team members and practicing nurses with information about the ongoing project. It was important to consider and include the ideas or thoughts of both groups.

Following the lead of the project initiator(s), participants made sure to consider each group's rights from an ethical perspective (e.g., a flexible schedule of meetings). Because the process was longitudinal and not always predictable, group members sometimes felt frustrated. It was important that the project leaders were patient, stayed in the here and now in partnership, and trusted in the transformative potential of a chaotic situation. Again, an appreciation of the theory was helpful in linking the dialogue to HEC. The participants learned to enjoy the evolving process, which was at times unpredictable and unidirectional.

Several strategies used in the project were consistent with the hierarchical culture of Japanese hospitals. First, we made an effort to foster an understanding and win agreement from the top level of the hospital's nursing departments about the intent of the project. These leaders then conveyed our invitation to the nursing units. Second, to provide continuity during the project, a head nurse and a nurse leader (e.g., a master's prepared nurse) were asked to be included in each group. It was the team's belief that the head nurses had a strong influence on staff nurses' motivation and therefore their inclusion in the group was crucial. Because head nurses were busy with unit management, the combination of head nurse and leader nurse worked well.

Phase 3: Identify a Hope Practicing Nurses Hold and Want to Actualize in Practice

At research/practice project meetings, dialogue was encouraged to identify a hope that the practicing nurses held and wanted to actualize in everyday practice. The hope was an image of desired nursing care. It was important to identify a hope and not a problem. As the hope is embedded in the nurses themselves, its actualization requires commitment of self and full involvement in the ongoing process. In contrast, a problem can be detached from the nurses themselves and be fixed instrumentally. Newman cited Morgan's description:

> When we engage in research action, thoughts, and interpretation, we are not simply involved in instrumental processes geared to the acquisition of knowledge but *in processes through which we actually make and remake ourselves as human beings.* (1994, p. 93)

Thus the process of actualizing a hope helps us make and remake ourselves as humans.

The participants at each meeting did not have any agenda for action. Instead, each participant, especially each practicing nurse, expressed a hope and actively listened to the others. This form of dialogue occurred over multiple meetings. As the participants who understood the theory interacted with other participants from the Newman theoretical perspective, pattern recognition occurred within the dialogue. Bohm (1990) believed that through the continuous participation in dialogue, a common mind can arise among the participants as they realize that the individual's hope, though it looks different, shares a common meaning. "If we could all share a common meaning, we would be participating together" (p. 15). In this project, the individual nurse's hope could become one with the hope of the unit nurses as a whole.

Within the project, the participants recognized their own patterns of thoughts, nursing actions, and ways of relating to clients through dialogue. For example, some nurses were aware of neglecting their relationships with the patients' families in everyday practice. One nurse realized her own care pattern as one of "doing" and not "being" with patients. Others discovered themselves as functioning only within a medical model of disease orientation. Through open and free dialogue, the participants began to talk as if they had known the theory from the beginning and expressed their own hope from an HEC perspective. Although their expressions were unique, all hoped to understand and help clients in the difficult situation of terminal cancer; at the same time, all hoped for their own growth as professional nurses. For each individual nurse, the various expressions of hope then became crystallized into a common hope—namely, to create a caring program with clients in the situation of terminal cancer in the framework of Newman's theory of HEC. Together, the entire team worked to apply the crystallization of hope as potential for action for this program.

Phase 4: Transforming Nurses' Hope into a Research/Practice Proposal

The clearer the "crystallized hope" was in participants' minds, the more feasible its actualization was in practice. Once the participants could fully imagine their own hope as nursing practice in reality, the next task was to transform it into a research/practice proposal. The team constructed a concrete image of the hope in the form of a pilot study. The dialogue between nurses and researchers continued throughout the process. The proposal was submitted to the hospital human subjects committee.

The nurses' group shared a draft of a caring program as a concrete expression of their hope at the group meeting. The first proposed "caring program" included a few opportunities for a primary nurse to have dialogue with a primary client, but was really more of a step-by-step manual of how to conduct an interview. This beginning attempt to model Newman's research guidelines was far from the essence of the theory of HEC. Soon the nurses realized that this approach was a reflection of their "usual" pattern of care. As the dialogue continued, the team began to focus on patients' and their families' situations, their needs, the nurses' primary responsibility, and caring from the theoretical perspective. This dialogue deepened the understanding of the essence of the theory. The proposed pilot study was modified, deleting many specifics of when, how, with whom, where, and why nurses would practice, allowing the nurses flexibility and creativity as they were inspired by the essence of the theory in the moment.

Phase 5: Putting the Proposal into Practice, Integrating It with Reality

Practicing nurses who volunteered to participate in the pilot study were asked to write reflective journals whenever they worked with the clients and to share them at the project meetings. Volunteer nurses put the proposed caring program into practice. Each nurse entered into partnership with a client and initiated a dialogue based on "the most meaningful persons and events in your life" (Newman, 1994, pp. 147–149). The nurse could modify this question to fit the client's particular situation. With their experience of the client–nurse partnership, the nurses described awareness, self-revelation, and changes in the way of they related with the clients through their journals. At the same time, they addressed some points that needed to be modified in the proposal.

While sharing the journals at the project meeting, nurses were invited to draw a simple diagram of patterns uncovered in the client–nurse dialogue on the blackboard. This was followed by dialogue among the participants, which facilitated pattern recognition in each team member along with the nurse who shared the journal. Pattern recognition was accompanied by expanding consciousness. In each instance, the participant had an opportunity to recognize her own pattern, the pattern of nursing care, and the pattern of relationships with clients. Pattern recognition led the participants to a realization of new rules of care, responsibilities, and ways of relating to clients. The mutual process among the participants was a meaning-making, transforming process. It was helpful for all participants to write in their own journals after each meeting.

The first presentation by one of the staff nurses was very exciting for the team. The nurse read her journal at the meeting, and all participants actively listened to her presentation. The journal was full of awareness, self-revelation, and transformation of self in the client–nurse partnership. A diagram of the client–nurse relationship pattern was then drawn on the blackboard. The changing pattern in the client–nurse relation was revealed vividly in the unfolding process. The nurse's pattern revealed a unidirectional relationship with the family, "looking to do something for them." One day, the family had approached the nurse and she took advantage of this opportunity. This process fostered a mutual relationship among all involved. When the nurse clearly recognized her pattern within the diagram, she experienced a transformation. She said, "I had thought this family understood nothing, but I recognized that the one who had not understood anything was me." The atmosphere of the meeting loosened suddenly. All participants were moved to tears and praised the nurse for her caring, considerate actions, courage, and transformation.

This nurse proposed a few points for revision in the program to better fit it with the clients' various situations in the terminal stage of life. Through dialogue, the caring program was modified so as to allow nurses more flexibility and creativity. The project team realized that these modifications facilitated commitment on the part of the practicing nurses in creating new client–nurse relationship model as well as enhancing practice wisdom.

Phase 6: Proposal Modification and Integration into Practice

As the project moved toward integration into practice, other staff nurses learned about it. From this group, other volunteer participants were invited to put the revised caring program into practice. They fully participated in the model of dialogue, reflection, and action and shared their experiences in integrating the caring program with the reality in the client–nurse partnership. This ongoing process continued to be repeated.

As transformations occurred, the practicing nurses' increasing awareness became apparent. When the participants were convinced of the benefits of the program to both the clients and themselves, it was felt that this research/practice project had reached the last phase. The nurses' hope continued to be actualized in everyday nursing practice.

Phase 7: Continued Action and Reflection

The revised caring program was modified at one more point. It was often not easy for young nurses to enter into partnerships with patients and their families. In this difficult situation, the nurses were sometimes experiencing chaos themselves. On these occasions, the head nurse or the leader nurse entered into partnerships with the young nurses and interacted with them to facilitate their pattern recognition. The project team found that young nurses who were helped by the expert nurses were then able to work with clients and to help them as they had been helped.

It took more than two years to reach the endpoint of the project. The actualized nurses' hope prevailed in the everyday nursing practice on the unit, and the ongoing process of nurses' transformations in care greatly influenced other nurses on units throughout the hospital.

Phase 8: Reporting Project Findings

The primary data from this investigation included the following sources: the practicing nurses' journals, which included their thoughts, feelings, awareness, and changes in ways of relating with clients; transcriptions of the tape-recorded dialogue at the meetings; other participants' journals; and the related descriptions in the nursing charts. In addition, other evidence dealt with implied enhancements in the quality of nursing care: clients' appreciations, bereaved families' expressions of gratitude, physicians' active responses to nurses, nursing students' positive appraisals, an increased caring atmosphere in the unit, and a decrease in staff turnover. These outcomes were used as additional data, as action research allows for the use of multiple data sources (Reason & Bradbury, 2000).

The focus of data analysis was the process underlying each practicing nurse's expanding consciousness and the similarities that emerged among them. Evidence of expanding consciousness included pattern recognition, awareness, self-revelation, and new ways of relating and acting in the process of unfolding transformation of self. With pattern as the basic assumption of the unitary, transformative perspective, the research team sought to identify the process of nurses' patterning as well as the clients' patterning within the context of the mutual process of the nurse–client relationship. Moreover, with the assumption that any pattern change emanating from practicing nurses spreads over the whole, further analysis may lead the team to identify the process in which the patterning of the project members facilitated the patterning of other staff nurses and other health providers.

Links to HEC

The praxis model of care and pattern recognition is neither simply reflective nursing practice nor simply nursing research. As Newman states, "the process of nursing practice is the content of nursing research" (1994, p. 92) when practicing in this manner. Newman's (1994) method of presentational construing of the data to portray evolving patterns over time for individuals and of the propositional construing of similarities within the group of individuals was effective in this study.

The research team portrayed the evolving patterns for each nurse practicing from a HEC theory base who worked with clients experiencing cancer— that is, the process of individual nurses' expanding consciousness. The resulting diagram helped the nurses gain insight into their patterns, find the action potential in care, and realize their own personal and professional growth. The team looked for similarities across the patterning of nurses, with general themes of transformation and portraying the sequential patterns. The process evolved through several phases: (1) What do I do and how?; (2) Who am I?; (3) recognizing pattern bounded in "should have to do"; and (4) moving on in partnership. This was the process of the team's expanding consciousness as a whole (Endo, 2000). All participants understood the meaning of the assertion that "our task was to fall toward the center of ourselves" (Newman, 1994, p. 101). Without this recognition, the nurses were afraid to relate to clients using Newman's theory. Following this personal recognition, they easily moved toward practice actions that enhanced the quality of their relationships with clients. This realization was enlightening to all.

Ethical Dimensions of the Project

To respect the privacy and confidentiality with clients, collaborators, and other staff, ethical sensitivity was an ever-present consideration. The team believed that to practice from this model generated an authentic caring presence in the nurse–patient relationship. To be authentic with any partner, Newman states, "we have to stand in the center of our truth. As we become able to center and to let go of boundaries, we will be able to create a vision of a caring community from which transformation will follow" (2003, p. 6).

Conclusions

This action research demonstrated that nursing praxis can make an important difference for collaborating practicing nurses and researchers and move them toward actualizing our hope in everyday activities of nursing. Newman's HEC theory provided a framework to guide both the research process and clinical practice. The outcome serves as a guide to individualize care and foster professional development.

References

Bohm, D. (1990). *On dialogue*. Ojai, CA: David Bohm Seminars.

Endo, E. (2000, June). *Hospital nurses' application of Newman's theory of health*. Poster presentation, Conference on Phenomenology and Hermeneutics, Minneapolis, MN.

Newman, M. A. (1994). *Health as expanding consciousness* (2nd ed.). New York: National League for Nursing.

Newman, M. A. (2002). The pattern that connects. *Advances in Nursing Science*, 24(2), 1–7.

Newman, M. A. (2003). The immediate applicability of nursing praxis. *Quality Nursing: The Japanese Journal of Nursing Education & Nursing Research*, 9, 188–190.

Reason, P., & Bradbury, H. (Eds.). (2000). *Handbook of action research: Participative inquiry & practice*. Thousand Oaks, CA: Sage.

CHAPTER FOURTEEN

RECOGNIZING PATTERNS IN THE LIVES OF WOMEN WITH MULTIPLE SCLEROSIS

JANE NEILL

Introduction

Recognizing pattern in individuals living with a chronic condition such as multiple sclerosis (MS) contributes to understanding the whole person. It allows for an appreciation of the illness experience and of how people respond to an array of unpredictable changes in life. Health as expanding consciousness (HEC) and its unitary, transformative philosophy brings personal and professional changes in practice, research, and education. This chapter applies Margaret Newman's theory in research and gives voice to what we know about pattern through the lives of women with MS.

The study from which this research is drawn took place in Adelaide, South Australia, and involved a two-year partnership with seven women, four of whom had MS and three of whom had rheumatoid arthritis (Neill, 2001, 2002a). A description of the life patterns and personal transformation for the women with rheumatoid arthritis, and an explanation of two underlying patterns for all the women, are given elsewhere (Neill, 2002b, 2002c). As reported here, the women with MS related detailed life stories containing narratives about their illness experiences. From these stories, both life patterns and underlying patterns were recognizable.

Relevant HEC Concepts

Understanding health as expanding consciousness for women living with MS reveals the pattern of the whole person, and elucidates how it is manifested in life patterns, underlying patterns, turning points, and choice points.

According to Newman, "learning to see pattern—to trace its unfolding transformation" (2002, p. 8) is fundamental to comprehending HEC. The *pattern of the whole person* interacting with the environment is apparent in our individuality, embraces order and chaos, and is indivisible from any illness (Newman, 1990, 1994). *Life pattern* can be seen within the personal story as manifestations of expanding consciousness unfolding in space/time. *Underlying pattern* represents what Bohm (1980) called the implicate order, or what Newman (2002) calls the ground of consciousness, and may also be seen in life stories. Underlying patterns are theoretical phrases evolving from contemplation of the meaning of individual and multiple life stories (Neill, 2001), although they do not depict the entire implicate order. Both life and underlying patterns help nurses appreciate people as unique, whole human beings.

HEC is described as evolving in seven stages, revealing increasing turmoil and chaos prior to a turning point, then restoration of order and personal growth (Newman, 1994). A *turning point* can represent a crisis, but it does not involve choice. For example, a diagnosis of MS can be a viewed as a personal turning point without choice. A *choice point* is identified by change, either sudden or gradual, which reestablishes a new order as people make intentional choices about new and more complex ways of living. Barrett's (2000) theory of power supports this idea. At the choice point, an individual is able to reclaim power as he or she participates knowingly in change. This is manifested by an awareness of possible choices, freedom to act intentionally, and involvement in creating change. Recognizing pattern with insight and subsequent change can result in greater complexity of the whole (Newman, 1994). This is more characteristic of choice points than turning points (Neill, 2001, 2002c). Examples of both are found in the women's stories.

Multiple Sclerosis

MS is a nonfatal, chronic condition affecting the central nervous system (CNS) that is seen two or three times more often in women than in men. The illness usually develops during early to middle adult life. Approximately 85% have a relapsing-remitting course rather than the rarer primary progressive, secondary progressive, or progressive-relapsing illness (National Multiple Sclerosis Society, 2003). Worldwide, an estimated 2.5 million people have MS. In 2001, approximately 15,000 Australians were living with MS (MS Australia, 2003). The prevalence of MS in Australia varies from north to south and is about 29 cases per

100,000 in South Australia (McLeod, Hammond & Hallpike, 1994). In the United States, a similar latitude effect is seen, with approximately 400,000 people being affected (National Multiple Sclerosis Society, 2003). MS is more common in people with northern European ancestry. Individuals with first-degree relatives affected by MS have a greater risk of developing the illness during their lifetime (Poser, 1994b). Although the cause of MS is unknown, its pathogenesis involves autoimmune inflammation of myelin, which covers the nerves in the CNS. This inflammation is followed by development of multiple sclerotic plaques and alterations to the blood–brain barrier (Poser, 1994a). Recently developed treatments such as Betaseron are aimed at modifying the immune response, reducing damage to the CNS, and limiting symptoms of the illness.

People Living with MS

Individuals living with MS report an array of unpredictable clinical symptoms, depending on the extent and location of damage to the CNS, making the disease difficult to diagnose. Most people do not develop severe disabilities (MS Australia, 2003). Nevertheless, the most disabling symptoms appear to be fatigue, heat intolerance, motor or sensory problems in limbs, loss of balance, and incontinence (Black, Grant, Lapsley & Rawson, 1994; Koch, Kralik, Eastwood & Schofield, 2001; Stuifbergen & Rogers, 1997). Pain, depression, and altered sexual identity also affect quality of life (Gilmore & Strong, 1998; Koch, Kralik & Eastwood, 2002; Sadovnick et al., 1996). Individuals living with MS cope with profound stress, symptom variability, diagnostic ambiguity, the knowledge that no cure exists, unpredictable exacerbations, and other people's reactions to disabilities associated with the illness (Antonak & Livneh, 1995; Koopman & Schweitzer, 1999). Gagliardi's description of the turmoil following her diagnosis of MS (Gagliardi, Frederickson, & Shanely, 2002) illustrates this stress.

Nursing research describing the experience of MS is increasing. The literature includes ethnographic interviews with war veterans about living with MS (Barton, Magilvy & Quinn, 1994; Quinn, Barton & Magilvy, 1995) and phenomenological descriptions of living with relapsing-remitting MS (Miller, 1997) or being diagnosed with MS (Koopman & Schweitzer, 1999). Participatory action research has shown how nurses can assist people to manage aspects of living with MS such as incontinence, sexual concerns, or hospitalization (Eastwood, Koch & Kralik, 2002; Koch & Kelly, 1999a, 1999b; Koch, Kralik & Eastwood, 2002; Koch, Kralik, Eastwood & Schofield, 2001).

Nursing theories also provide useful interpretive frameworks for understanding the experience of living with MS. A study using Roy's theory of adaptation (Gagliardi, Frederickson, & Shanely, 2002) involving 18 people with MS identified five themes of change in people's lives consistent with Roy's four adaptive modes. Data showed that each person experiences MS and its effects on his or her quality of life differently. Comprehensive assessment by nurses using Roy's theoretical model is a useful framework for nurses to understand responses to adapting and changing lifestyles for patients experiencing MS. Understanding individuals' experiences with MS can also be enhanced through pattern recognition and HEC.

One study used aspects of HEC to interpret the experience of living with MS for women. Using Heideggerian hermeneutics, Koob, Roux, and Bush (2002) described inner strength as five constitutive patterns consistent with Newman's view that disease is a manifestation of (underlying) pattern. Similarities were evident between the patterns describing inner strength and the underlying patterns in the study described here. Koob et al. (2002) however, asked phenomenological questions about inner strength, rather than unitary questions about pattern such as: "What are the life patterns (person–environment interactions) of women living with MS?" and "What patterns of the whole person can be discerned from women's life stories?" (Neill, 2001). The following discussion provides an understanding of life patterns and underlying patterns in women living with MS.

The Women in This Study

Four women living with MS—known as Rose, Margaret, Helen, and Sarah—volunteered to share their stories about living with MS. These participants ranged in age from 44 to 58 years and following diagnosis had lived with MS from 5 to 18 years. All lived independently with community support. Rose, Helen and Sarah had full-time, live-in caregivers who were also their male partners. Margaret had a part-time caregiver female friend. Each had one to four children and had been single parents for part of their lives. Margaret was adopted as a child and had recently located her birth family. She and Helen were born in Australia, whereas Rose and Sarah were immigrants from the United Kingdom. All were of white, northern European ancestry. None had been educated past middle to upper secondary school level, but all had worked in clerical positions, manufacturing, or service industries. None had been financially secure during their early lives, and all were now receiving disability pensions. Rose and Sarah still worked as volunteers.

Rose had known about her diagnosis of relapsing-remitting MS for only five years. At the start of the study, she was considering whether to begin Betaseron treatment. Eventually she decided on treatment but had difficulties with the side effects of the medication.

Margaret had lived with relapsing-remitting MS for 18 years, and had recently developed a secondary progressive course. After each relapse, she noticed further functional losses and felt depressed about being a "good" grandmother.

Helen had lived with undiagnosed symptoms since her late adolescence before discovering she had relapsing-remitting MS while in her early forties.

She faced daily uncertainty with unpredictable episodes, and was hospitalized the previous year for a severe exacerbation.

Sarah had primary progressive MS, which she described as "downhill since day 1." She needed a wheelchair for mobility, but grieved the loss of feeling in her hands more acutely than losing her balance. Although she realized her MS was progressing, Sarah remained confident that she would be around for another decade or more.

Pattern Recognition Process

Newman's research protocol (1994) was used to recognize pattern during nursing partnerships with the women. Up to four in-depth, unstructured interviews were held with each participant over a two-year period. These interviews involved recounting life stories featuring important people and events the participants remembered; recognizing life patterns; reflecting on meaningful photographs taken by the women; and reviewing our partnerships and the study before closure (Neill, 2001, 2002a, 2002b, 2002c). Narratives from the women's stories were arranged in chronological order, allowing individual life patterns to be identified; underlying patterns were seen as recurring themes across life pattern. The study ended after each woman received a draft of her life-pattern story and gave her response to it (Neill, 2002c). Details of each interview, analysis, and interpretation are reported elsewhere (Neill, 2002b).

Life Patterns of Women Living with MS

Table 14.1 summarizes the life patterns for the four women. Rose and Margaret had similar life patterns, beginning with happiness, becoming vulnerable, struggling to regain self, and finding new ways of living with MS. But the people and events in their stories were unique. Helen and Sarah had dissimilar life patterns, but neither remembered consistent happiness or feeling good about herself as a young person. Lifelong issues of power and control were evident in their stories and patterns.

Underlying Pattern Representations

Each of the women had three of five identifiable underlying patterns recurring through her life pattern (Table 14.2). These underlying patterns are theoretical phrases representing complex phenomena. They emphasize a process involving movement and change, rather than the categorical meaning of words

Table 14.1. LIFE PATTERNS OF FOUR WOMEN LIVING WITH MS

| | DEVELOPMENTAL STAGE | | | | | |
	CHILDHOOD	YOUTH	YOUNG ADULT	MID-LIFE	LATE ADULT	OLDER AGE
Rose	Happiness and protection	Being vulnerable and overcoming exploitation	Struggling to regain self in the face of loss	Finding new ways of being		
Margaret	Happiness with friends and family	Surviving the cruel blows of life	Struggling to regain self	Finding purpose in life		
Helen	Control: conflict and chaos			Release: change and choice		
Sarah	Being silent		A decade of chaos	Speaking out		

Table 14.2. UNDERLYING PATTERNS IN THE LIFE PATTERNS OF FOUR WOMEN WITH MS

| | UNDERLYING PATTERNS | | | | |
	ENERGY~FATIGUE	GIVING~RECEIVING	VULNERABILITY~RESILIENCE	CONTROL~RELEASE	BEING SILENT~SPEAKING OUT
Rose	Primary	Secondary	Accessory		
Margaret	Primary	Accessory	Secondary		
Helen	Primary	Accessory		Secondary	
Sarah	Primary	Accessory			Secondary

used. The primary and secondary patterns were most distinct, with accessory patterns being less prominent.

The underlying patterns of "energy~fatigue" and "giving~receiving" were noticeable in all of the women's stories. Brief exemplars of how these patterns were manifested are given elsewhere (Neill, 2002b, 2002c). The way these underlying patterns were expressed resembles Newman's early proposition about a fusion of apparent opposites, disease and nondisease, in a meaningful concept of health (Newman, 1994). In addition, these theoretical phrases expressed the evolving pattern of the whole person, in that the first descriptor's meaning dominated the women's early lives, but after a choice point usually occurring around mid-life, the second descriptor's meaning prevailed. For example, having and using plenty of energy, giving to others, vulnerability, control of or by self or others, and silence were characteristic of the women's lives before a choice point. Afterward, the women learned new ways of living with fatigue, receiving help from others, being resilient to loss and change, gaining release from control over their lives by others, or speaking their own truth.

The Women's Stories: Life Patterns, Underlying Patterns, and HEC

Life patterns and underlying patterns are revealed in the women's stories, as well as turning points, choice points, and the process of expanding consciousness. Each story has been abbreviated and should be read in conjunction with Tables 14.1 & 14.2.

Rose's Story: "Whatever You Give, You Receive"

The earliest of four life patterns provided happiness and protection, whereby Rose learned that "whatever you give, you receive" and recognized the value of working hard to achieve this goal. In a second life pattern as a young person, Rose left her protective family by marrying and immigrating to Australia but felt vulnerable and exploited as people took advantage of her giving nature. When her husband abandoned her just before their son's birth, Rose felt most isolated and vulnerable. With motherhood, she became more assertive. Some years after her divorce, she met her second husband and joined Al-Anon, a support organization for families affected by alcohol addiction. Al-Anon gave Rose "a roadmap for life" and helped her deal with alcohol, food, and work addictions in her family.

As a young adult, Rose felt her life was becoming increasingly disordered. Early signs of MS were discounted as trivial. Then Rose was hospitalized with an acute episode that confirmed the diagnosis. She struggled with loss after discovering she had MS but tried to "take life into her own hands" again. The spiritual relationship she developed with her "higher power" and supportive friends in Al-Anon also helped. When she returned to employment, fatigue and numb fingers affected her work.

Rose's turning point was being laid off from a job she loved because of her MS. While she was devastated by the loss, her choice point involved becoming a volunteer. Volunteering allowed her to conserve energy for valued activities and enjoy work again by giving and receiving. Rose found new ways of living with MS, became firmer about saying "No," and maintained her connections with others and with her higher power. Rose's story shows the importance of reciprocity in giving to and receiving from others and the value of support.

Margaret's Story: "Still Me Inside"

Margaret was adopted as an infant and enjoyed a happy life with her mother, sister, stepfather, and friends in her first life pattern. Her happiness persisted until after her marriage and the birth of her children. When her husband was transferred to another state, a life pattern of vulnerability emerged. During this time, Margaret spent enormous energy on fitness and family commitments, and she experienced considerable turmoil. She survived a cyclone and lost her home, and she endured the death of her mother, her husband's unfaithfulness and emotional abuse, her friend Lyn's diagnosis of cancer, and emergence of her MS. For a while Margaret believed she was "going nuts" because her symptoms were not validated by a diagnosis for eight years. During this period, she discovered great resilience in times of vulnerability. Following a "stroke-like" collapse at work soon after the end of her marriage, she was diagnosed with MS.

Margaret coped with the impact of MS by "changing everything" about her lifestyle, forming new connections especially with her birth family, regaining her sense of humor, and becoming "tougher." Eventually she could no longer work or manage daily living without help, and she considered herself to be a burden on her adoptive family. Margaret's choice point involved returning to the city from a remote area, to independent living, with Lyn as her part-time caregiver. In her most recent life pattern, Margaret formulated goals for what was important, and she found ways to help others.

MS had affected Margaret profoundly. As she said, "My body is stuffed, I know that. But inside, I feel like a million dollars." Elaborating on this paradox, she explained, "Because I'm still me inside, and I like the way I am. I'm happy with myself." Margaret's story shows how she developed resilience from great vulnerability and recognized her own resources.

Helen's Story: "I Didn't Listen to My Body"

Helen's early life pattern persisted until her middle age, a time full of disorder and disruption. In this pattern, she was controlled by others, or was attempting to gain control of self or others. This led to conflict and prolonged chaos in Helen's life. During mid-life, she finally acknowledged the MS that had begun in her early adulthood. Before this turning point, Helen felt that her life was out of control. She managed a family of four children; worked full-time, and kept going "past the pain barrier" so she rarely slept properly. Helen also endured abuse from her mentally ill husband, as well as the deaths of her brother and father, before MS compelled her to recognize the limitations imposed by her lifestyle.

Helen's choice point involved leaving her marriage and trying to come to terms with many changes. The emotional barriers that she had constructed to protect herself left her feeling "numb," and it was a long time before she could enjoy life and laugh again. After the choice point, Helen's life pattern heralded many changes. Being released from her previous pattern of control allowed her to emerge from the chaos and conflicts of the past. Living with MS also helped Helen develop new awareness about her body, which tended to "shut down" unexpectedly, leaving her unable to speak or move. If she set limits and heeded her body instead of ignoring its limitations, she was less likely to lose control of her speech and movement. She explained, "I mean I *know* what my body's telling me, I just didn't listen. And your body does talk to you if you listen." During a severe exacerbation of MS, when she felt she might die, Helen realized that she could trust God to get her through anything about life with MS. Her story reveals her struggle to change the balance of control in her life and to gain new respect for her body.

Sarah's Story: "Just Ignore It—and It Will Go Away"

Sarah's early life and first life pattern were dominated by silence, which led to lack of choice, difficulty with decisions, and making sacrifices for others. Silence about problems or illness gave a superficial appearance of harmony in her family. "It must be the British upbringing, and 'stiff upper lip.' You know, ignore it and it'll go away." During this first life pattern, Sarah tried to extricate herself from family control when she became an adolescent mother. When her husband insisted they immigrate to Australia, Sarah vacillated but then accepted his decision in silence.

In her second life pattern, Sarah endured a decade of chaos, marked by sacrifices, silences, and deferred decisions, yet the family and cultural pattern of reserve kept Sarah silent when she needed to speak out. At the end of this decade, during which her mother died, her brother committed suicide, her father died after surgery for cancer, and her husband abandoned her and two young children, Sarah was diagnosed with primary progressive MS. At the time, she worked seven days to support her children, and maintained silence about the traumas she had faced. In spite of her symptoms, Sarah tried to ignore what was happening, as she felt unable to make decisions to change her exhausting lifestyle. She remembered thinking, "I developed MS and that was it! The decision was made for me."

Consistent with the pattern of progressive MS, Sarah made choices to change her life gradually. The emerging life pattern was distinguished from her past experiences by breaking her silence in many ways. For years, Sarah could not mention the devastating events in her life, but participating in this research study gave her an opportunity to do so. Sarah's story revealed how she paid more attention to her remaining abilities, overcame silence, and emerged as a strong advocate for others with MS.

Health as Expanding Consciousness

While Rose and Margaret began their lives in happy family environments, Helen and Sarah felt that control issues made their early years less than ideal. Nevertheless, all of these women found their lives becoming chaotic with the loss of people, relationships, work, or traumatic events. They identified turning points that provided impetus for change, and all except Sarah, who made more gradual changes, reached clear choice points where they made

decisions about their futures as women living with MS. Choice points initiated a process of personal transformation expressed as transcendence of self,
space, and time (Neill, 2002b). While Koob et al. (2002) believed expanding
consciousness began with a life event such as the diagnosis of MS, this study
of four women with MS revealed that expanding consciousness occurs
throughout a person's life in continuous movement toward greater complexity, as Newman's theory explains.

Underlying patterns were manifested during each unfolding life pattern in
different forms for the women, but the pattern of the whole person was expressed more harmoniously when they found new ways of living with MS that
restored order to their lives. Two of these new ways, *finding simple pleasures* and
being positive, have also been described for women living with rheumatoid
arthritis (Neill, 2002b). Two additional new ways of living for the women with
MS were *self-control* and *self-differentiation*. They felt in control of their illness, and
perceived themselves as whole beings, separate from their illness. Inner
strength, as Koob et al. (2002) describe it, was evident in how the women
changed their lives by reclaiming control, solving problems in different ways,
and gaining new perspectives on themselves and illness.

Photographs Reflecting Pattern and Expanding Consciousness

After sharing their life stories, the women continued their reflections by taking
photographs using a small disposable camera. At the third interview they
selected some photographs to share in discussion, and they gave additional
consent to allow reproduction of these images. Photographs have been used
to illuminate the meaning of various health and illness experiences, because
they provide symbolic expression of intimate meanings about phenomena
(Hagedorn, 1994, 1996). Although no single image conveyed all that was meaningful to the women, each photograph depicted important people, places,
and feelings. Interpreting the images was a hermeneutic process, intertwining
personal meanings, life patterns, and underlying patterns.

Mostly the women photographed other people, pets, landscapes, or still
life images. Three had photographs taken of themselves. The main themes in
Rose's photographs were the simple pleasures she gained from the natural
world and making gifts for others, which reflected her underlying pattern of
"giving~receiving." Margaret shared photographs of her grandson's birth and
the football players she supported, which symbolized her ways of being
positive and finding simple pleasures. Helen shared photos of her partner,
their pets, and their favorite places, which signified her inner strength in living
with MS. An image of her three dogs perched together in Helen's wheelchair
(see Figure 14.1) symbolized her acceptance of and control over her illness,

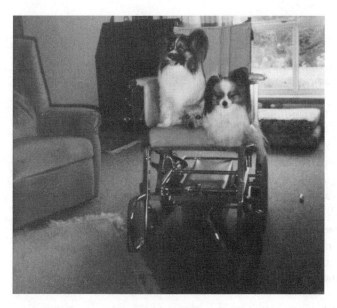

Figure 14.1. Helen's wheelchair symbolized her new self-control, and the dogs were her "reason to get up each day."

and she described the dogs as a reason to get up each day. Sarah's photographs depicted peaceful and beautiful corners of her house and garden, representing her underlying patterns in its new manifestation of appreciating silence by choice, and her ability to differentiate self from illness. Each photograph taken by the women seemed to illustrate an aspect of their patterns and the meaning of health as expanding consciousness.

Conclusions

This chapter illustrates how nurses can give voice to what we know about Newman's theory of HEC through research. Recognizing the pattern of the whole person is a form of caring and is the way we come to know others (Newman, 2002). Life patterns, underlying patterns, turning points, and choice points can be recognized when a life-story dialogue evolves within a caring nursing partnership. This "caring praxis" (Neill, 2002c) entrusts nurses to be with people experiencing upheaval in their lives, as they find insights and make intentional choices about change. All of the women with MS had difficulties before this study began, but the process of telling their life stories and recognizing patterns helped them reconcile their past lives with their present selves. Developing partnerships of caring praxis and recognizing the pattern of the whole person transforms research endeavors through health as expanding consciousness.

References

Antonak, R. F., & Livneh, H. (1995). Psychosocial adaptation to disability and its investigation among persons with multiple sclerosis. *Social Science and Medicine*, 40(8), 1099–1108.

Barrett, E. A. M. (2000). The theoretical matrix for a Rogerian nursing practice. *Theoria: Journal of Nursing Theory*, 9(4), 3–7.

Barton, J. A., Magilvy, J. K., & Quinn, A. A. (1994). Maintaining the fighting spirit: Veterans living with multiple sclerosis. *Rehabilitation Nursing Research*, 3(3), 86–96.

Black, D. A., Grant, C., Lapsley, H. M., & Rawson, G. K. (1994). The services and social needs of people with multiple sclerosis in New South Wales, Australia. *Journal of Rehabilitation*, 60(4), 60–65.

Bohm, D. (1980). *Wholeness and the implicate order*. London: Routledge & Kegan Paul.

Eastwood, S., Koch, T., & Kralik, D. (2002). Compromising and containing: Self-management strategies used by men and women who live with multiple sclerosis and urinary incontinence. *Australian Journal of Holistic Nursing*, 9(1), 33–43.

Gagliardi, B. A., Frederickson, K., & Shanely, D. A. (2002). Living with multiple sclerosis: A Roy adaptation model-based study. *Nursing Science Quarterly*, 15(3), 230–236.

Gilmore, R., & Strong, J. (1998). Pain and multiple sclerosis. *British Journal of Occupational Therapy*, 61(4), 169–172.

Hagedorn, M. (1994). Hermeneutic photography: An innovative esthetic technique for generating data in nursing research. *Advances in Nursing Science*, 17(1), 44–50.

Hagedorn, M. (1996). Photography: An aesthetic technique for nursing inquiry. Issues in *Mental Health Nursing*, 17(16), 517–527.

Koch, T., & Kelly, S. (1999a). Identifying strategies for managing urinary incontinence with women who have multiple sclerosis. *Journal of Clinical Nursing*, 8(5), 550–559.

Koch, T., & Kelly, S. (1999b). Understanding what is important for women who live with multiple sclerosis. *Australian Journal of Holistic Nursing*, 6(1), 14–24.

Koch, T., Kralik, D., & Eastwood, S. (2002). Constructions of sexuality for midlife women living with multiple sclerosis. *Journal of Advanced Nursing*, 39(2), 137–145.

Koch, T., Kralik, D., Eastwood, S., & Schofield, A. (2001). Breaking the silence: Women living with multiple sclerosis and urinary incontinence. *International Journal of Nursing Practice*, 7, 16–23.

Koob, P. B., Roux, G., & Bush, H. A. (2002). Inner strength in women dwelling in the world of multiple sclerosis. *International Journal for Human Caring*, 6(2), 20–28.

Koopman, W., & Schweitzer, A. (1999). The journey to multiple sclerosis: A qualitative study. *Journal of Neuroscience Nursing*, 31(1), 17–26.

McLeod, J., Hammond, S., & Hallpike, J. (1994). Epidemiology of multiple sclerosis in Australia. *Medical Journal of Australia*, 160(163), 117–122.

Miller, C. M. (1997). The lived experience of relapsing multiple sclerosis: A phenomenological study. *Journal of Neuroscience Nursing*, 29(5), 294–304.

MS Australia. (2003). MS *Information*. Retrieved May 6, 2003, from
http://www.mssociety.com.au/msinformation/.

National Multiple Sclerosis Society. (2003). *About* MS. Retrieved May 2, 2003, from
http://www.nationalmssociety.org/about%20ms.asp.

Neill, J. (2001). *"Broken into wholeness": Life patterns of women living with multiple sclerosis or rheumatoid arthritis*. Unpublished PhD Thesis, Flinders University, Adelaide, Australia.

Neill, J. (2002a). "Broken into wholeness": Life patterns of women living with multiple
sclerosis and rheumatoid arthritis. *Rogerian Nursing Science News Online*, 1(2), [2p].

Neill, J. (2002b). Transcendence and transformation in the life patterns of women
living with rheumatoid arthritis. *Advances in Nursing Science*, 24(4), 27–47.

Neill, J. (2002c). From practice to caring praxis through Newman's theory of health as
expanding consciousness: A personal journey. *International Journal for Human
Caring*, 6(2), 48–54.

Newman, M. A. (1990). Newman's theory of health as praxis. *Nursing Science
Quarterly*, 3(1), 37–41.

Newman, M. A. (1994). *Health as expanding consciousness* (2nd ed.). New York, NY:
National League for Nursing.

Newman, M. A. (2002). Caring in the human health experience. *International Journal for
Human Caring*, 6(2), 8–12.

Poser, C. M. (1994a). Notes on the pathogenesis of multiple sclerosis. *Clinical Neuroscience*, 2(3–4), 258–265.

Poser, C. M. (1994b). The epidemiology of multiple sclerosis: A general overview.
Annals of Neurology, 36(Supplement 2), S180–S193.

Quinn, A. A., Barton, J. A., & Magilvy, J. K. (1995). Weathering the storm: Metaphors and
stories of living with multiple sclerosis. *Rehabilitation Nursing Research*, 4(1), 19–27.

Sadovnick, A., Renyck, R., Allen, J., Swartz, E., Yee, I. M. L., Eisen, K., et al. (1996).
Depression and multiple sclerosis. *Neurology*, 46(3), 628–632.

Stuifbergen, A. K., & Rogers, S. (1997). The experience of fatigue and strategies of self-
care among persons with multiple sclerosis. *Applied Nursing Research*, 10(1), 2–10.

PART FOUR
EDUCATION

CHAPTER FIFTEEN

PRAXIS AS A MIRRORING PROCESS: TEACHING PSYCHIATRIC NURSING GROUNDED IN NEWMAN'S HEALTH AS EXPANDING CONSCIOUSNESS

CAROL PICARD

TARA MARIOLIS

Introduction

The purpose of this chapter is to describe the mirroring of nursing praxis with nursing students as a way for them to experience, appreciate and understand the value of meaning and pattern in supporting health as expanding consciousness with the chronically mentally ill. Recent trends in nursing education and psychiatric care gave the authors pause to reflect and create a new teaching-caring model for baccalaureate nursing students.

Psychiatric-Mental Health Nursing and Education: Where Are We Going?

The past decade of psychiatric research has been mainly focused on the brain, with advances in technology contributing to an increased emphasis on neurobiology for answers to the problem of mental illness. Flaskerud and Wuerker (1999) emphasize the importance of a neuropsychiatric focus for mental health nursing. Although the contributions of research in molecular biology, genetics and psychopharmacology have led to a fuller understanding of these disease

Reprinted with permission from *Nursing Science Quarterly*, 15(2), 118–122. Copyright 2002 by Sage Publications.

processes and therapies, this knowledge cannot explicate the lived experience of living with a chronic mental illness. The day-to-day life of a person with a major mental illness has changed very little in the past 25 years. The chronically mentally ill live in the community and continue to feel marginalized in a society that does not understand them (Hall, 1997). They are still in need of caring nurses and other health professionals who will inquire: What is it like to live with your illness? and What holds meaning for you? The chronically mentally ill do need the latest in psychopharmacologic discoveries, but they are also in need of understanding.

Qualitative research studies examining the lived experience of the mentally ill have identified concerns related to quality of life. Perese (1997) found that the most frequently cited unmet needs of the mentally ill related to quality of life: friendship, role and purpose, membership in a group, and self-identity. The experience of feeling stigmatized marginalizes the person's experience of living. Vallenga and Christenson's study (1994) of persistent and severely mentally ill clients' perceptions of their mental illness identified that distress and suffering were in large part socially constructed by the community and institutions on which clients relied. The source of the distress was the stigmatization, alienation, and loss associated with having the illness.

A Caring and Learning Model for Clients and Students: Mirroring Praxis

The quality of life and wellness project was developed to provide a creative approach to learning based on a discipline-specific theoretical and philosophical base, and to address the concerns of the chronically mentally ill. This project involving baccalaureate nursing students, clients, and faculty was conceived of as a way to provide a care opportunity for clients and introduce students to care that was not based on crisis intervention and symptom management. The project, located on the college campus, was offered both to students and clients as a meaning-based nursing model of care to complement the traditional care services available in the area. An overview of the program itself is reported elsewhere (Mariolis and Picard, 2002). Both authors worked with clinical groups of six to eight students. Every week each student met with a client individually, and then the clinical group of students, their clients and their faculty member would come together for an hour-long group meeting with them later in the week. Students rotated every nine weeks, whereas the clients agreed to participate for two semesters at a time. Each client had the opportunity to meet with three students during the course of the year.

A Model of Praxis

Praxis according to Newman (1999) is a "deliberate, synchronous action and reflection involved in transformation" (p. 229). The faculty envisioned the project as praxis, where all involved—including the authors, students and clients—would have an opportunity for transformation through the appreciation of pattern. Newman's (1994) definition of nursing was "caring in the human health experience . . . manifested in a sensitivity to self, attention to others, and creativity" (pp. 139–140). Our belief was that mirroring a praxis mode of caring with students and clients would be reflected in the students' mode of being with clients.

Philosophical and Theoretical Ground: Roach and Newman

The writings of Roach (1992) formed the philosophical basis for the project and Newman's theory of health as expanding consciousness was central to the faculty's living of caring (Newman, 1994, 1999). Caring is defined by Roach as the human mode of being, and nursing was the professionalization of this capacity grounded in theory, research and clinical skill. The ontology of caring is what the nurse embodies and lives in his or her practice. Roach (1992) identified five attributes of caring. Compassion is defined as the ability to connect with and appreciate the experience of the other. Competence includes all the requisite knowledge and understanding necessary to the nursing situation and the concerns of clients. The attribute of confidence provides the patient with the nurse's attitude of assurance that they will be cared for. Conscience is the reflective ethical comportment of nursing practice and commitment is the ability to live up to one's practice of caring. These attributes guided faculty in the project's development, and we worked to shape an environment in which these attributes could be cultivated in students. As we lived these attributes with our students, we believed they could mirror them with their clients.

Newman's (1994) theory of health as expanding consciousness was relevant to teaching and learning about the care of the mentally ill. Newman drew from Rogers' science of unitary irreducible human beings to construct a theoretical framework of health as expanding consciousness. Every person is a consciousness, and has a unique pattern of wholeness manifested in movement, space and time. Pattern, according to Newman (1999), is a unique manifestation of the whole. "Pattern is a dynamic relatedness to one's environment, both human and non-human" (p. 228). As persons recognize their pattern, they have an opportunity for growth through insight as potential for action (Litchfield, 1999). Transcendence is the experience of moving to a higher level of consciousness, which is expressed in more meaningful relationships and greater sense of personal freedom (Newman, 1994). The capacity for self-reflection, self-expression, and self-understanding is an aspect of expanding consciousness. Nursing care can support a person's self-awareness. By appreciating the person's rhythm of relating to his or her world, and being fully present to hearing stories of meaning, nurses support the development of insight as potential for action. Newman (1994, 1999) believed that nursing is praxis, where the nurse embodies the theory. Through the process of self-reflection, the faculty and student nurses in this project learned to first appreciate their own pattern of expanding consciousness as preliminary and ongoing work to care for the clients in the project. The faculty created an environment to support the students' inquiry into and appreciation of their own pattern.

Newman has credited the work of Reason (1993) for his model of cooperative inquiry. This project was a form of cooperative inquiry into wellness and learning processes. Reason reflected that human inquiry is sacred science where knowledge must be a path to heal alienation, not simply to search for truth. Human inquiry is participative, where we engage with what we wish to understand. To teach nursing as caring in the human health experience, as defined by Newman (1994), faculty brought the weight of creative theory-based approaches to student learning.

The faculty members discussed core values that they wished to embody and live during the development of the model of care and teaching. First, they wanted to foster the cultivation of a capacity to be fully present to others, students and clients. They also believed in the essential wholeness of all students and patients, and valued each person's expression of wholeness as a unique and unrepeatable pattern. They hoped to invite students to see their clients as whole, and not through the lens of deficiency, as Hall (1997) described the current mainstream model of psychiatric care. The client's wholeness and potential for growth would be the anchoring beliefs of the project. The faculty also believed that change and growth is possible for all, including themselves, and could be supported by the caring presence of another. Both faculty spent considerable time sharing with each other and reflecting alone on their teaching approaches how to tailor approaches to student learning needs.

Mindfulness and Presence

The faculty used strategies to support a praxis mode of becoming in nursing. Newman (1994) suggests cultivating mindfulness, or a centering period, as a component of preparing for nursing practice. Faculty maintained a centering practice in this project to focus more mindfully on students and clients. Both faculty members had experience in different forms of mindfulness meditation. A mindfulness practice supports the capacity for being fully present to others. Presence involves focusing one's attention fully on the other. In living this process with their teachers, nursing students learned firsthand the experience of someone else being fully present to them. Before each meeting with clients, the students would participate in a mindfulness period of 10 to 15 minutes, focusing on the breath followed by a focused intention on assisting the clients that day. Although some students had experience with a mindfulness practice, for most it was a new experience. After each exercise, students were invited to reflect on the process of centering mindfully. Dialogue with their peers often included their concerns and desires to find a way to meet their clients' needs for connection.

Meaning and Pattern: Invitation And Exploration

The faculty members kept journals as the project began to reflect on the project. They also met with each other to discuss their own feelings as well as their understanding of the students and clients involved in the project. The students also kept journals, which provided an opportunity for them to explore anxieties about their own mental health and their fears about serious mental illness. They also used their journals to reflect on their patient's pattern of relating. They were invited to share their reflections, to the degree they chose, with their clinical group, as did the faculty members. They also had the opportunity to meet with the teacher individually on a weekly basis. Early in each rotation of students, the faculty posed the following question to the students: "What is most meaningful to you?" Students would respond in a variety of ways to this self-reflective exercise.

Boxes of Meaning: Self Exploration

One example of a self-reflective exercise was an invitation for students to bring a box to clinical seminar. In the box they were invited to place objects symbolic of what was most meaningful to them. In the seminar, they shared the contents with each other and the meaning of each item. Students frequently included pictures of their loved ones (deceased and living), pets, and symbols of valued parts of their lives such as athletic prowess, group affiliations, or the desire to be excellent nurses. In one group, the students' parting gift to the faculty member was to give her a box with a symbol of each one of them. Students shared that reflecting on meaning was an important exercise in getting to know themselves and each other. For some students, telling their story generated insight into their own patterns of relating. They appreciated the need for self-reflection when caring for their patients and could see the value in meaning based activity for clients as well.

In group discussions with clients, students were able to bring their unique talents and resources to offer as a part of enhancing quality of life. One student, who was also a musician, brought her flute to the group one week and played a meditative piece, which greatly impressed the clients. They expressed their appreciation at the opportunity to hear this other expression of her voice.

Expanding Imaginal Margins: Pattern Appreciation

Bunkers' (1999) conceptualization of the teaching learning process, based on Parse's human becoming theory, held similar values of honoring the other, as Newman's (1994, 1999) and Roach's (1992) work. As part of the student process of becoming, we as teachers were guides for expanding what Bunkers(1999) called their "imaginal margins" (p. 227). This expanding of imaginal margins involved entertaining a wider array of possibilities for understanding another. Both authors reflected on the unique responses and patterns of their students. In dialogue together, faculty discussed how to honor each student's unique contributions. Some students came with a great deal of life wisdom, and others were still new to the world of suffering and alienation in their clients' stories. Frequently, students had no experience with the mentally ill and were confronting their own stereotypes as they began the clinical experience. Although most nurses encounter patients when there is some disturbance in patterns of relating, the chronically mentally ill often have an increased sensitivity to the environment and its potential to disrupt their patterns. The expertise of the instructors in recognizing these patterns helped students to appreciate the intended meaning, and expand their imaginal possibilities for engaging their clients. Particularly in the beginning of each rotation, students often had difficulty seeing the patient as whole, often focusing on behaviors, which by society's standards, are considered eccentric or unusual. They did not understand the clients' rhythms of relating. Awkwardness was sometimes a mutual process for patients and students as they tried to establish the rhythm of their relationship. The imaginal realms of the students expanded through reflective dialogue with each other, their faculty member, and their client, as well as readings from nursing, and literary sources on mental illness. One of the authors referred to O'Brien's (1974) children's book Mrs. Frisby and the Rats of NIMH, to encourage sensing pattern. The book's main character finds that she needs courage to solve the challenge of rescuing her children. She is assured that she could unlock any door—all she needed was the key. When students were challenged by clients' use of language in unusual ways, faculty members would help students to imagine language differently, to find the key to appreciating the symbolic value or metaphorical intent that a person with schizophrenia, for example, might be struggling to express. The authors worked to help students to see that figuring out the key to understanding would enrich their patterns of relating. This placed the emphasis on the nurse's learning rather than a client deficit.

For example, one client who was extremely anxious upon meeting the group of students for the first time exclaimed that she was a famous country and western singer and that she didn't recognize where she was. The authors believed the client's reference to a famous singer perhaps expressed not only her own anxiety but her experience of the students' anxiety in the room as well. Faculty were quickly able to capture the meaning behind the words that the client was not feeling at home with newness of the program, the students or the faculty. Students could witness this interactional process and participate in conversation with the client about their newness as well.

As students planned activities with clients for the group sessions, they chose to mirror similar ways of exploring meaning with their clients: They introduced mindfulness exercises and invited clients to bring in photographs of themselves or those whom they cared about. They brought the clients journals for writing reflections and invited creative expressions in poetry and singing, accepting each person's contribution to planning of projects. Frequently, food was a part of the project, and students and clients would bring in something to share. Students were able to enhance their appreciation of the client's pattern of connecting, and they worked with that rhythm. One client, who had periods in which she felt disconnected from her environment in what she described as a dreamlike state, was helped by particular grounding techniques she and the student identified together.

Environment and Meaning: The College Campus

The campus is infused with meaning for the students. It is their temporary home. The clients were their guests on campus. The students discussed how they felt about their professional and personal worlds meeting. They had to consider how to respond to situations that would not arise on a hospital ward. For example, one student was unsure how to introduce her client to other students when they went for coffee, so she asked the client how she would like to handle this. The collaborative emphasis challenged traditional role relationships, similar to Byrne's (1999) description of pubic health nurses' change in perspective about power relationships in their work with the chronically mentally ill in empowerment groups. The project required an attitude of partnership. The campus environment was infused with meaning for clients as well. The clients were not defined by their illness in this space or marginalized in social interaction in this space. The energy on a college campus is filled with a rhythm of class schedule times, movement of large numbers of students every 50 minutes, and an emphasis on learning, and becoming. On the first day the project began, the clients remarked on how excited they were to be in college. They were quick to point out, however, that they knew they were not official students, but that they had enrolled in the project to learn something new. Several clients shared how they always wanted to go to college but their illness got in the way. The "imaginal margins" (Bunkers, 1999, p. 27) of the clients expanded as they claimed this public college as part of their personal community geography. They were excited to learn with the students and to have time to explore the campus and use the facilities.

Appreciating Client's Pattern

Meeting for 9 weeks in this project allowed each student to come to know his or her client in a unique way. Spending 2 hours each week focusing on well-being and meaning allowed them to have a different sense of the client's pattern than they would have had in an acute care setting, focusing on symptom management. Each student and client reflected together on how to shape what the project could offer them and made a commitment to work together. For some, this meant simply to be in dialogue each week. Other clients wanted to use the campus facilities to exercise. Some used the library, game room, and cafeteria. Students and clients would participate in these activities together. Another client who valued her femininity, wanted very much to enhance her grooming. The student working with her brought in makeup and together they engaged in learning to apply the makeup. Clients and students identified personal goals as part of the project. Although some clients dropped out of the program because of challenges with being organized to get to the campus regularly, there were others who surprised their case managers by faithfully attending, despite tremendous difficulties with episodes of their illness, logistics of transportation, and lack of self-organization skills. They expressed a valuing of the program in their determination to participate.

Students were able to articulate their appreciation of the person they were caring for and could see the bigger picture of the context of their story, relationships, the importance of meaning and the influence of mental illness in their clients' lives. Students were also in contact with their client's other care providers in the community whose agenda may have had a similar goal, but whose focus was medical and behavioral management. Students could appreciate the efficacy of medications but continued to see beyond the disease to the person and their day-to-day living. An important part of this experience was appreciating and honoring their client's patterns of relating, however unique and idiosyncratic.

Appreciating Student's Own Pattern

The students who participated in the care model became more aware of their own patterns of relating. Reflection and engagement taught this lesson as one of the students, Jan DiNatale (1999) shares below. Most of the baccalaureate students in this clinical experience will not go on to be psychiatric nurses. However, they will provide health care to the mentally ill, and have a greater appreciation for the person beyond the illness. They will also be better informed to educate nurses who are reluctant to care for the mentally ill in other healthcare settings. Their care reflected competence, confidence, compassion, conscience and commitment (Roach, 1992) to this group of clients.

The following are excerpts from a journal entry by DiNatale (1999) at the closing of her practicum experience with this project:

> Tuesday was an awesome day. Several of us played cards in the cafeteria and had a great time. All clients were thinking clearly, with connected speech patterns, rational communication, emotionally stable. There were no tears or disjointed thoughts. We acted as a group, worked on our task, card playing, and enjoyed each others' company- all our psychosocial needs were met. (The group had gone to an exhibit of modern art that day in the campus gallery.) It's interesting to note their response to the art exhibit. They all thought it quite strange, didn't care for it much. They had the chance to see that art is an individual perception and it's OK not to like it. I didn't care much for it myself. This is an excellent opportunity for student nurses to interact and come to know clients with schizophrenia in the community milieu as opposed to a crisis environment. It opens your eyes to the wonderful and delightful spirit within us all, something we are born with. To experience joy and acceptance in ourselves and others, is, to me, the meaning of life. We need it to live as much as we need oxygen. I think very few of us have enough love in our lives because the world can be a rather loveless place. So this coming together is good for all of us.

Conclusion

The chronically mentally ill can benefit from nursing care that emphasizes pattern appreciation and quality of life. This approach attends to their concerns for meaningful connection and group membership; it supports a sense of self-identity beyond illness. By considering new environments for caring and learning in the community, faculty can support and enhance quality of life for those living with mental illness. A caring-based model of teaching-learning is a way to mirror praxis for students as they develop themselves in nursing. Grounded in nursing theory, this type of model is discipline-specific and expands the imaginal realm of students to see clients beyond a symptom management perspective and through a nursing lens of wholeness. Faculty can mirror praxis for students in their clinical experiences through the student-faculty relationship. Through the experience of a mindfulness practice, presence and pattern appreciation can be cultivated.

References

Bunkers, S. S. (1999). The teaching–learning process and the theory of human becoming. *Nursing Science Quarterly*, 12 (3) 227–231.

Byrne, C. (1999). Facilitating empowerment groups: Dismantling professional boundaries. *Issues in Mental Health Nursing*, 20 (1), 55–72.

DiNatale, J. (1999). *Clinical reflections*. Unpublished manuscript, Fitchburg State College, Fitchburg, MA.

Flaskerud, J., & Wuerker, A. (1999). Mental health nursing in the 21st century. *Issues in Mental Health Nursing*, 20 (1), 5–18.

Hall, B. (1997). Looking at chronic mental illness through new trifocal lenses. *Journal of the American Psychiatric Nurses Association*, 3, 27–30.

Litchfield, M. (1999). Practice wisdom. *Advances in Nursing Science*, 22 (2), 62–73.

Mariolis, T. & Picard, C. (2002). The quality of life and wellness program: A model for teaching psychiatric nursing care. *Journal of Nursing Education*, 41 (11), 501–503.

Newman, M. A. (1994). *Health as expanding consciousness* (2nd Ed.). New York, NY: National League for Nursing.

Newman, M. A. (1999). The rhythm of relating in a paradigm of wholeness. *Image: the Journal of Nursing Scholarship*, 31 (3), 227–230.

O'Brien, R. (1974). *Mrs. Frisby and the rats of* NIMH. New York, NY: Atheneum.

Perese, E. F. (1997). Unmet needs of persons with chronic mental illnesses: Relationship to their adaptation to community living. *Issues in Mental Health Nursing*, 18, 19–34.

Reason. P. (1993). Reflections on sacred experience and sacred science. *Journal of Management Inquiry*, 2(3), 273–283.

Roach, S. (1992). *The human act of caring*. Ottawa: Canadian Hospital Association.

Vallenga, B. A. & Christenson, J. (1994). Persistent and severely mentally ill clients' perceptions of their mental illness. *Issues in Mental Health Nursing*, 15, 359–371.

Chapter Sixteen

Cultivating a Way to Sense Pattern with Advanced Practice Nursing Students

Hollie Noveletsky-Rosenthal

Kathleen Solomon

Introduction

Teaching nursing students using a framework grounded in Newman's (1994) theory of health as expanding consciousness (HEC) presents challenges and opportunities. The authors used a model of structured reflection with graduate nursing students to promote pattern appreciation in both students and clients. Links between HEC and the teaching strategy used are presented here as well as student responses to the process. The authors used new strategies to assist students in uncovering a nursing identity.

Professional Identity and HEC

Graduate-entry into nursing is a relatively new educational model in the United States. Students in these programs enter nursing preparation after having already earned academic degrees in other fields. This model presents unique challenges to the professional acculturation of students. Traditionally, the development of a professional identity for undergraduate nursing students occurs over time through the process of socialization as a student, then as a novice registered nurse. In contrast, graduate-entry students enrolled in accelerated programs to sit for licensure at a midway point in the curriculum, and then graduate as advanced practice nurses experience a different process of socialization. The development of a professional nursing identity is a challenge particularly as these students enter the advanced practice component of the curriculum. These challenges include having non-nursing mentors or preceptors, taking on a nursing role that shares a substantial knowledge base in medical science and many tasks with medicine, and a mixed and inconsistent use of nursing knowledge within a clinical practice environment.

A critical step in the development of the nursing student's professional identity is the ability to identify and voice a nursing perspective that differentiates his or her practice from that of other disciplines. Newman, Sime, and Corcoran-Perry (1991) believe that nursing's unique perspective is grounded in its focus on the human health experience. Within the framework of HEC, health is defined as one's pattern of relating to the environment, and the focus of practice is to understand the evolving nature of the individual's pattern (Newman, 1994). Newman developed a practice-research method to uncover the individual's pattern through the use of the narrative.

To uncover the meaning embedded within another's story, the student must be present to the individual. Reflective practice cultivates this skill. By incorporating guided reflection into clinical nursing education, students can develop a greater ability to be present to their clients, and to grasp the meaning of each client's health experience. This approach can provide students with an opportunity to appreciate the unique nursing role of the advanced practice nurse and to use the HEC focus to understand more fully the human experience.

The concept of pattern is central to HEC (Newman, 1994). The pattern of the individual reflects an implicate or underlying order and is manifested through interactions with his or her environment over time. This implicate order represents the essence of the individual, his or her way of being in the world. Within the framework of HEC, pattern is unique to each person. During the course of their dialogue, the nurse and the client are able to experience the present by also reflecting on the past. The ability to grasp a full understanding of pattern is gained by appreciating the past, the present, and the potential for the future. One's pattern is uncovered through a reflective process of examining multiple interactions over time and looking for recurring themes or ways of interacting. Pattern evolves over time. Patterns of interaction that limit the individual from connecting with the environment can block the individual's ability to engage and evolve to higher levels of consciousness (Noveletsky-Rosenthal, 1996). Movement toward higher levels of consciousness is manifested through a richer quality of interactions with the environment. The nurse and the client engage in a mutual process during the unfolding dialogue. Both client and nurse patterns can hinder or enhance the ability to connect with each other (Newman, 1999). Therefore, it is essential that nursing students uncover their own patterns of interacting so that they can cultivate their capacity to be fully present to their clients.

Prior to undertaking this project, the authors believed that advanced practice nursing students focused significant energy on becoming technically proficient in the provision of care. During their educational experiences, they often missed opportunities to see the evolving patterns emerging from the interaction between the clients and themselves. At times, students experienced difficulty in establishing therapeutic relationships with clients and were unable to identify why such problems occurred. As faculty, we saw the potential to enhance therapeutic relationships and assist students' recognition of the nursing contribution to the health experience of their patients.

Structured Reflection

Johns' model of structured reflection is a middle-range theory consistent with HEC (Johns & Freshwater, 1998). The model was developed to assist novice nurses in their professional development by uncovering their own tacit knowledge base and to help them move along the continuum from novice to expert. This evolution from novice to expert nurse is consistent with Newman's theory of evolution of consciousness. As a nurse or student gains knowledge they develop a greater appreciation of the whole clinical experience through an ability to integrate a broader quality and range of knowledge simultaneously (Benner, 1984). Similarly, within the framework of HEC, as a person evolves toward higher levels of consciousness, he or she is able to integrate a broader quality of information manifested through a deeper level of connectedness with the environment (Newman, 1994).

Johns (2002) encourages self-reflection as a way for students to uncover their own pattern of interaction. Reflection is essential for developing insight into pattern, and for learning new ways of interacting. Insight and choosing ways of interacting are congruent with Newman's processes of pattern recognition and pattern transformation. Pattern recognition can assist in a student's professional role development as well as support his or her interaction with clients.

The reflective practice model (Johns & Freshwater, 1998) offers students multiple lenses, or framing perspectives with which to view their interactions. Using these lenses, students have the opportunity to uncover factors that they bring to the interaction and to recognize how these factors might influence the quality of the relationship. As they examine multiple interactions over the course of a semester, patterns of interaction emerge. Within the framework of HEC, the pattern of the individual is uncovered. However, no structure is provided for the telling of the narrative. Johns' model does offer such a structure. In advanced practice nursing education, there is an emphasis on the learning and integration of standard clinical data; Johns' model helps the student look beyond the data to develop a more holistic appreciation of the encounter.

Within the educational preparation of the nurse practitioner, there is a covert valuing of the medical model. Case presentations based upon a medical diagnosis and treatment have become widely accepted as a teaching method in graduate nursing programs. Students are often taught to present cases according to this model. Such an approach restricts the student's perspective to examine the significant aspects of the clinical encounter. Johns' reflective model, using multiple lenses as tools to encourage taking a broader perspective of the interaction, facilitates the process of pattern recognition.

There are eight framing perspectives in John's model:

1. Philosophical framing
2. Role framing
3. Theoretical framing
4. Parallel pattern framing
5. Problem framing
6. Reality framing
7. Temporal framing
8. Framing the development of effectiveness (Johns, 2002; Johns & Freshwater, 1998)

While these framing perspectives do not capture the whole of the interaction, they do invite the students to look at subtle factors that they bring to the interaction and that help shape its quality.

Through the lens of *philosophical framing*, students clarify "ideal" practice. They examine personal beliefs and values regarding the nature of person, life, and practice as they relate to the provision of "ideal" care. The *role framing* lens focuses students' examination of the issues of professional boundaries, relationships, and power. Through the lens of *theoretical framing*, they identify the theoretical and scientific knowledge necessary to provide "ideal" care. The lens of *parallel pattern framing* allows students to recognize the dynamics of interaction through role-play. In addition, they are able to explore alternative ways of interacting to enhance their ability to connect with clients. The lens of *problem framing* directs student learning toward uncovering and clarifying the covert and sometimes subconscious issues that affect the quality of interactions. *Reality framing* helps students to understand how context influences an interaction's quality and outcome, while the lens of *temporal framing* gives students an opportunity to appreciate the evolving nature of pattern.

Consistent with the theory of HEC, students come to understand how their past experiences influence their present interactions and become incorporated into new experiences that shape their future interactions. Through the lens of *framing the development of effectiveness*, students learn to value reflective learning within their own evolving patterns of interaction (Johns & Freshwater, 1998; Johns, 2002).

In addition to these eight framing perspectives, Johns (1997a, 1997b) developed reflective cues to assist students in the reflective practice process. These cues consist of pointed questions to help direct students into a deeper level of self-reflection. Examples of the type of questions Johns developed are, "What was I trying to achieve [in the interaction]? Why did I respond as I did? . . . How did I feel in this situation? What factors embodied within me or embedded within the environment were influencing me?" (Johns, 1998, p. 4). These cues assist the students in moving beyond a superficial analysis of an interaction toward a deeper and more holistic appreciation of the experience.

Reflection as Process

The advanced practice clinical seminar is a time for students to integrate theoretical preparation and clinical practice. Often clinical seminars become a place to learn from the experiences of their peers. Our seminar group consisted of nine advanced family practice nursing students in a graduate-entry program. They were engaged in various primary or ambulatory care clinical settings. The seminar group was scheduled to meet weekly for two hours and was based on Johns' model. During the seminar, students were expected to share clinical experiences and present clinical situations. In addition, they kept weekly journals of their clinical experiences and received written feedback on their journal entries from their seminar leader.

Each individual in the group processed information and interacted with patients differently, and the faculty worked with each learner to respect these differences while providing a safe and supportive environment for the process of self-reflection to occur. This interaction and support was critical to the process. Students expressed the importance of being able to openly discuss their experiences with the faculty and classmates and receive feedback from their classmates. The faculty created a protected environment to allow this process to occur. They encouraged collective reflection, respected each individual's perspective, and established seminar confidentiality. Once safety and openness for dialogue were established, the process of engagement and reflection accelerated. Students were motivated and eager to gain a deeper understanding of self so as to provide better client care. Learners discovered how to connect with clients in the brief encounters within clinical practice. The students came to value those opportunities as the essence of their practice and understood that it was the connection established with each patient that separated their practice from that of other professionals. One student commented:

> There are many times throughout my clinical days where I find myself wondering how it is possible that I am allowed to listen to another person discuss with me intimate details of his life. It is often in the patient's discussion about his journey with or through illness that the character of his being is illuminated. It is in *this* adverse moment when he becomes true to himself. So I continue to sit here and ponder how fortunate I am to bear witness to such a moment of discovery.

Another student reflected on the value of what is *not* said in the clinical encounter:

It is valuable to reflect on the unspoken exchange that occurs in the exam room because there is so much that is communicated in nonverbal ways. Those are the things that are so helpful to think about.

At the end of the semester, students reviewed weekly journal entries in chronological order to examine and reflect on their own personal and professional growth. The authors conducted a thematic analysis of each journal. Over the course of the semester, specific themes began to emerge for the students. These centered on addressing situations where the students' personal values came into conflict with the values of their clients. Students also described becoming aware of their personal biases in areas related to abortion, forms of abuse, smoking, and teen sexuality. Other themes included being present to another, personal anger, honesty, patient disclosure, professional relationships, and communication. Recurring themes were then examined in light of student insight and manifestations of pattern recognition. The authors found that students were able to gain insight into their own patterns of interaction, and reevaluated personal beliefs and actions to reduce self-imposed barriers to connecting with clients. One student's journal reflected this insight:

I guess the lesson I learned for today is the importance of these small details. And although I may sometimes feel that the time I spend with a patient might be better spent discussing more relevant matters, in the end, what becomes meaningful is exactly what the patient decides to share with me.

The termination process for the seminar group was difficult. The group had developed into a connected and supportive unit. Through the process of collective and individual self-reflection, the participants came to know themselves, one another, and the seminar leader with a deep level of understanding. The group process was a manifestation of the evolution of consciousness of both the individuals and the group as a whole. Because of this deeper knowing, the process of separation became more difficult. To sustain their connections with one another, the students developed an Internet-based dialogue group.

Discussion

This use of HEC and structured reflection enhanced the students' ability to actively focus on clinical practice. Reflection *on* practice is the foundational stage of self-reflection (Johns & Freshwater, 1998). During the process one learns to retrospectively reflect on his or her actions. As the nurse moves from novice to expert, he or she develops the skills of reflection *in* action.

Reflection in action is the ability to reflect on a situation while in the midst of the experience. It represents a more advanced level of self-reflection due to the simultaneity of the processes of reflection and action.

Johns' model includes the assumption that a nurse's practice should continually strive to approximate ideal care through ongoing learning and self-discovery. It provides a structure for evolving self-awareness and invites a deeper understanding of values, beliefs, and ways of interacting. Reflective practice also provides a framework for novices to begin to uncover their tacit knowledge, which Benner (1984) said marks the journey from novice to expert. Tacit knowledge must be developed and nurtured, and is the dialectic product of science and perceiving. The model developed students' ability to simultaneously integrate actions with their knowledge base to know the experience as a whole. Grasping the whole is a distinguishing characteristic of the expert and the HEC-grounded nurse.

Integration of Reflective Practice into Advanced Nursing Practice Curriculum

Self-reflection is an essential nursing competency in advanced practice education. It provides a strategy to integrate theoretical, scientific, and personal knowledge to ground quality care, and is consistent with a caring perspective and Newman's theoretical framework of HEC. Other forms of knowledge take their rightful place within the advanced nursing practice learning process, but the nurse–patient relationship is the central focus of practice. While this project was conducted with graduate-entry advanced practice students, it is equally relevant for all nursing students, regardless of their educational level or point of entry. The authors believe the best place for inclusion of reflective practice strategies in the curriculum is in the clinical seminar. This can be enhanced through practice and journaling.

Conclusions

As technology in health care advances, the need to maintain caring connections with patients remains fundamental. Advanced practice nurses are in a unique position to reach out and establish these connections with people at their most vulnerable times. Reflective practice provides a means for strengthening students' ability to grasp the meaning of health for each client. Teaching HEC with reflective practice strategies to advanced practice nursing students offers an opportunity to discover a true nursing identity. As one student summarized, "Once again, it's a situation in which I cannot physically *do* much. However, emotionally I can offer an infinite amount of compassion and support. This is why I love nursing."

References

Benner, P. (1984). *From novice to expert*. Menlo Park, CA: Addison-Wesley.

Johns, C. (1997a). Reflective practice and clinical supervision—part 1: The reflective turn. *European Nurse*, 2(2), 87–97.

Johns, C. (1997b). Reflective practice and clinical supervision—part 2: Guiding learning through reflection to structure the supervision "space." *European Nurse*, 2(3), 192–204.

Johns, C. (Ed.). (2002). *Guided reflection: Advancing practice*. London: Blackwell Science.

Johns, C., & Freshwater, D. (Eds.). (1998). *Transforming nursing through reflective practice*. London: Blackwell Science.

Newman, M. A. (1994). *Health as expanding consciousness* (2nd ed.). New York, NY: National League for Nursing.

Newman, M. A. (1999). The rhythm of relating in a paradigm of wholeness. *Image: Journal of Nursing Scholarship*, 31(3), 227–229.

Newman, M. A., Sime, A. M., & Corcoran-Perry, S. A. (1991). The focus of the discipline of nursing. *Advances in Nursing Science*, 14(1), 1–6.

Noveletsky-Rosenthal, H. T. (1996). *Pattern recognition in older adults living with chronic illness*. Unpublished doctoral dissertation, Boston College, Boston, MA. Dissertation Abstracts: University of Michigan.

CHAPTER SEVENTEEN

DOCTORAL STUDENT EXEMPLAR: TRANSFORMATION OF THE PATIENT–NURSE DYAD

SUSAN M. LEE

Introduction

Students work with theory, which they learn in a classroom or read from a textbook. The real challenge is to use the theory in practice and apply principles and concepts embedded in a theoretical position to guide clinical practice. After reading about the unitary-transformative paradigm and discussing the perspectives of Newman, Rogers, Watson, and others, I made a conscious effort to look at my practice more critically, evaluate my interaction with patients, and seek new opportunities that fostered the links between theoretical positions and actual practice. The exemplar given in this chapter reflects a conscious effort to accomplish this goal. At the conclusion, I will summarize the advantages of theory used to guide practice from the perspective of the student and offer some recommendations for consideration by clinicians and educators.

A Critical Care Exemplar: Transformation of the Patient–Nurse Dyad

Ask a nurse to recall a memorable patient, and he or she will often relate the drama of an emergency, the satisfaction of early problem recognition, challenging patient or physician behaviors, or a situation in which the nurse-patient relationship was particularly rewarding. In the archives of our memories are stories of patients who changed our thinking, our practice, and nurses as human beings.

Exemplars have been used by Benner (1984) and others to explicate embedded nursing knowledge in practice. In this chapter, an exemplar is seen as a rich source of cognitive and affective dimensions within the nurse–patient relationship. It represents a beginning attempt to explicate caring behaviors that are so taken for granted in nursing that they may be even more difficult to elucidate than embedded knowledge. Noddings (1984) said that it is easier to justify our actions and give a rationale for them than to articulate what motivates us and touches us. In addition, a question posed by Newman, Sime, and Corcoran-Perry will be answered: "What is the quality of the relationship that makes it possible for the nurse and the patient to connect in a transforming way?" (1991, p. 35).

First Night

I wasn't assigned to Cathy on her first night in the coronary care unit (CCU). There were two nurses on duty, and my partner took her. "She looks like hell," commented a 3–11 nurse. "I've never seen her look so bad."

I remembered her name and remembered her being in the unit before. I wasn't sure about her story except that she was labeled a brittle, type 1 diabetic and that she had a reputation of being an "actress" and a "drug addict." She was also known to complain of chronic chest pain. She was "most comfortable" titrated up to the maximum level on intravenous (IV) nitroglycerin without batting an eyelash.

"Frequent flyers" are what we called them, the chronically ill who became part of our community hospital family. We knew them well, their families, and their stories. Cathy was particularly tough. She was 45 years old.

Cathy had been discharged from the hospital just 24 hours earlier following the surgical debridement of foot ulcers. After arriving home, she began to experience vomiting and diarrhea and was encouraged by her visiting nurse to return to the emergency room (ER) for evaluation. She presented at the ER with fever and a question of sepsis. IV fluids were given for volume depletion.

I saw her around midnight trying to climb out of bed. The monitor cables, oxygen tubing, IV tubing, and Foley catheter were tangled and stretched to their limits. I rushed in to prevent her from falling. She threw her arms around my waist and hugged me like a frightened child. I put my arms around her and held her against me. She was dyspneic and tachypneic and throwing her legs over the side of the bed—classic behaviors associated with patients in pulmonary edema. I let her stay wrapped around me and listened to her back— "crackles all the way up to her neck."

"It's okay. We'll help you. Looks like you had a little too much fluid in the ER. I hear fluid in your lungs. It's just some water and we can pull that right out with some Lasix." She let go and put herself back into bed.

Cathy had been a diabetic since her teenage years. The disease resulted in many functional changes, such as retinopathy, neuropathies, peripheral vascular disease with amputations of five toes, a femoral-popliteal bypass, coronary artery disease that won her eight cardiac catheterizations and three angioplasties, constant chest pain, gastroparesis with a J-tube at one time, and foot ulcers. She had numerous hospitalizations with us and had also been frequently sent to tertiary care facilities.

Paradigmatic Perspectives

Newman, Sime, and Corcoran-Perry (1991) suggested that all nursing research has been conducted from one of three paradigmatic perspectives that range from physical to social to human science. The paradigms are named by hyphenated terms. The first component of each refers to the entity being studied; the second component refers to the process of change.

Particulate-Deterministic Paradigm

The first paradigm, the *particulate-deterministic* perspective, considers phenomena as isolated, measurable entities. The process of change is viewed as linear and causal. Identifying antecedents is a first step to prediction and control. Knowledge is accepted only if it is verifiable. Located within this perspective are Aristotelian views of knowledge as objective and observable. Perspectives derived from this point of view include positivism, objectivism, rationalism, and reductionism. Physical processes amenable to measurement, such as serum cortisol levels or glucose levels, are used to support veritivity when conducting research within this paradigm. Nursing research usually involves the health of the body as affected by environmental factors (Newman, 2000).

Interactive-Integrative Paradigm

The second paradigm, the *interactive-integrative* perspective, is an extension of the particulate-determinate perspective. Within this perspective, concepts are viewed as multidimensional and contextual. Although the perspective still involves prediction and control, subjective data are legitimately used to understand phenomena of concern, demonstrating a move toward holism. This perspective cannot be considered truly holistic, however, because the analysis of person is still carried out in a particularistic way with the goal of knowing the patient through the sum of the parts. "The prevailing paradigm assumed that it was valid to analyze human beings into parts, reduce those elements to measurable entities, control and manipulate the parts, and try to extrapolate to the whole based on knowledge of the parts" (Newman, 2000, p. 81). Although it is consistent with post-positivism, evidence within this perspective suggests that a shift is occurring toward ontological knowing and value placed on multiple ways of knowing. Nursing knowledge is derived by observation as well as report, history, family, and other contextual cues. Nursing research within this paradigmatic perspective looks at the interplay of body-mind-environment factors in health.

Unitary-Transformative Paradigm

The third paradigm is a unique, emerging perspective, not evolving from the first two. The *unitary-transformative* perspective considers a phenomenon as a unitary, self-organizing field embedded within a larger, self-organizing field. Distinct from previous linear, causal paradigms featuring multidirectional change in isolate entities, change in fields is unidirectional, moving toward more complex organization. Inquiry within this paradigm involves pattern recognition by both the viewer and the subject in a process of mutuality and unfolding. The unitary-transformative paradigm rejects prediction and control as being integral to nursing practice. Instead, pattern is viewed as the identifying characteristic of a person's wholeness.

The uniqueness of person is reflected in the moment, and manifestation of wholeness is reflected in the interaction of person and environment. The nurse engages in this experience and his or her intentional presence helps uncover truth and foster personal choice.

Linking Theory to Practice

The particulate-deterministic perspective is dominant in critical care. Knowledge is derived from observation, physical parameters, and technology. The patient's subjective knowledge is considered legitimate only if it can be verified or objectified, for example, on a pain scale.

In "First Night," the nurse hears stories of a "difficult patient" whose veracity and authenticity are questioned by other nurses. Nurses share personal stories reflecting their perceptions of experiences with patients. Sometimes in a "one-upmanship" style, a nurse recounts an experience—for example, "I've got a better one than that." Before nurses care for patients, expectations and biases are formed. Judgments about the patient are made, the nurse's ability to connect with the patient is compromised, and ethical care is jeopardized. When the nurse bases care upon others' perceptions of the patient, the nurse begins to care holding a priori beliefs of the patient that affect her assessment and subsequent care plan. An example relevant to Cathy might be that the nurse, holding a priori beliefs that Cathy was an "actress" would not immediately medicate her for pain because the nurse believed that Cathy was not experiencing physical pain.

In "First Night," assumptions within the particulate-deterministic perspective are evident—for example, in the form of Cathy's chest pain. Nurses did not see her complaints of chest pain as legitimate because the symptoms were reflected verbally and subjective knowledge is not recognized in this paradigm. In addition, Cathy's chest pain was not verified because tests for coronary artery disease were always negative, and nitroglycerin would have alleviated it, if the problem were physiologically based. Interestingly, it was not then widely known that neuropathy could be a cause of chest pain although Cathy did have gastroparesis, another form of neuropathy. When viewing symptoms within the medical paradigm, a search for causality dominates.

As a result of this perspective, all phenomena without verifiable evidence are considered not to exist, including all subjective responses. What does this mean to the patient when all experiences, thoughts, feelings, and symptoms not substantiated by evidence are seen as not legitimate? This perspective can devalue a person as a feeling, sentient being. The particulate-deterministic perspective is limited and views a person as a physiologic process. It has the least application in nursing science where person is valued for all he or she is at a point in time. Within the dominant paradigm, this perspective is self-perpetuating within the critical care community. Each new member is acculturated to the paradigm, and the existing community cannot conceive of it being any other way (Newman, 1995).

The particulate-deterministic paradigm in the intensive care unit is a powerful shaper of nursing care. Veteran nurses do not willingly recognize or accept other paradigms. They focus on "physiologic stability" first. While appropriate, it can limit the person's participation in care.

An alternative is reflected in the behavior of the nurse who was not assigned to Cathy in "First Night." When Cathy reached out for the nurse, the nurse responded in a human way, reaching back for the patient which manifested caring, being with (presence), and taking in the wholeness of the person beyond the illness. The nurse was reassuring. By not pushing her back in the bed, but by taking time to comfort and assess, the stage was set for the caring relationship that ensued. "I know what to do and I am here for you." Cathy's dyspnea and fright prompted her to reach out. This was the antecedent for the nurse to act in an intentional way, become engaged, and give of herself in meaningful presence so that both the giver and the receiver were edified (Nelms, 1996). Therefore, the stage was set for a mutual, transformative process that has been called the essence of nursing (Newman, 1995).

Day 2

The next day, Cathy was intubated after a respiratory arrest. Bilateral pneumonia was the medical diagnosis. I cared for her during the evening hours. Her husband interrupted shift report repeatedly: "Cathy needs pain medicine. Cathy wants to be suctioned. Cathy wants ice chips. Cathy wants to change position. Cathy needs the bedpan."

"Cathy would be fine if her husband would go home," said the nurse going off duty. "I tell him, 'Go get a cup of coffee, Jim,' and that gets him out of here for a while. I've known Jim a long time. He takes care of the patient and their daughter who is wheelchair-bound. I haven't been out of that room for 12 hours." The nurse was exasperated. I wondered how many cups of coffee Jim had drunk and how that contributed to his anxiety.

I introduced myself to Cathy and Jim and reviewed my plan for the evening. They were agreeable. Jim was giving Cathy a backrub. She was sitting up in bed with the ET tube hanging from her mouth. Her vent settings and readings told me she was very comfortable. The tube was clear without secretions. A head-to-toe assessment, partial bed bath, change in position, and Demerol followed. Although I always allowed family to stay, Jim's presence was distracting to Cathy. I shut out the lights and Jim turned off the TV. "Let's give her a rest anyway, Jim," I said softly.

The Dynamics of Care

In critical care, the clipboard flow sheet, with its multitude of blank boxes, can dictate nursing care. Time permitting, "other" care is given, ranging from less crucial tasks such as shaving the patient to interpersonal interventions such as educating and supporting the family. Newman puts it this way, "The explication of knowledge relevant to caring in the human health experience is affected by paradigmatic perspective" (1995, p. 39). Therefore, how we view a person determines the care we give.

In "Day 2," the nurse is beginning to "come to know the patient as person." The evaluation of physical function by reviewing the vent settings suggests physical comfort. Vent settings and readings are some parameters used in the overall patient picture to determine comfort. But by addressing only physical parameters to evaluate health, there is a fragmenting of body, mind, and spirit. The "whole" is minimized and functional health presupposes in this case "total comfort."

Knowing the Person

Knowing the patient is considered a central concept in nursing practice, an "immediate grasp" and "directly apprehended" (Tanner, Benner, Chesla & Gordon, 1993, p. 275). In a review of nursing literature, Radwin (1996) found that knowing the patient means understanding the patient and being able to determine the correct interventions. Knowing the patient is "getting a grasp of the patient, getting situated, understanding the patient's situation in context with salience, nuances, and qualitative distinctions" (Tanner et al., 1993, p. 275). The concept is relevant across paradigms, although how the nurse accesses and receives knowledge and responds with interventions will yield different outcomes.

Knowing the patient within a HEC perspective offers the patient the opportunity to be known as the focus of inquiry, and seeks to have a story be told by the participant from his or her perspective. Within the partnership with the nurse, the patient reveals himself or herself. In the shared process, a dynamic exchange occurs between nurse and patient. In the end, both are affected by the presence of the other.

Nights 4 and 5

The next time was a bit easier. With Cathy still vented but with Jim now at home, I cared for Cathy on the 11–7 shift. "To increase your comfort and let you get some sleep, I have a plan. Let me know what you think. We'll do everything in clusters like turning and suctioning and backrubs and vital signs. Then, I'll give you the Demerol, and I'll let you sleep until you wake up. I will be in the room puttering. I'll replace the cold cloth on your head, and I won't let you go more than two hours without Demerol. I will just give it to you, okay? The call bell will always be on your belly button. If ever you can't find it, just take the pulse oximeter off and the machine will alarm and I'll come running."

Cathy gave me the thumbs up sign. For three consecutive nights, we were a team. She trusted me and knew that I would not leave the room until everything was done to her satisfaction. I told her every blood pressure, lab result, every positive step she made. She was always aware of her progress and it looked like she would be weaned any day.

"If that tube doesn't come out today, I won't mind," I told her one morning. "We're getting lots of stuff out now. The pneumonia's breaking up, and we're able to go right down and get it outta there. So, don't be too disappointed if today is not the day. There are benefits to keeping it in." She nodded.

Links to Knowledge and Practice

In "Nights 4 and 5," the nurse describes an evolving relationship with Cathy that includes many affective, cognitive, and temporal elements, manifested as a synchronous whole. While the whole is more than the summative parts, elements will be discussed separately here to show the complexities of the patient–nurse dyad. The *temporal* aspect of the relationship, now three consecutive nights, gave the nurse the time to "know the patient." The nurse *knew* the patient's preferences and needs as well as physiologic parameters that provide evidence of comfort—for example, low peak inspiratory pressures, amount of secretions in endotracheal tube, clear breath sounds, and physical appearance such as ability to rest and sleep. These achievements were gained through continuity, knowledge, and intentional presence of the nurse.

"Nights 4 and 5" represents a culminating point in the nurse–patient relationship. The exemplar illustrates the relatedness of the nurse and the patient in a dynamic interplay. Although it is difficult to reduce the relationship to its subelements, some are explored here to provide evidence of the transforming nurse–patient dyad. Noddings' (1984) terms of the one-caring and the one-cared-for will form the basis of the discussion.

The nurse as the one-caring brings an attitude of care, a receptivity to what is there, "as nearly as possible without evaluation or assessment" (Noddings, 1984, p. 34). Newman (2000) describes it as an unconditional acceptance of the client's life pattern over time. The nurse has discarded all preconceptions of the patient and entered into a relational mode or receptive mode, which forms the basis of the caring relationship. Boykin and Schoenhofer (1993) assert that this attitude is necessary for the fullest form of nursing knowledge where the nurse is living grounded in caring. The ICU nurse must continue to assess empiric data in an analytic-objective mode. However, there is a conscious and fluid movement observed between the analytic mode and the relational or receptive mode (Noddings, 1984). The nurse has discovered situations and practices that afford the patient comfort. A routine or a series of tasks performed in a certain manner provides security and communicates care to the patient. The nurse engages in tasks with a caring attitude that says, "I care about you and I will do these things that are important to you. I know you are fearful. I hear you and I will respond to you." The mere physical presence of the nurse in the room and the purposeful reassurance that the patient will not be left until mutual goals are achieved connote care and respect of personhood. The nurse shows concern for the patient's well-being by communicating in ways such that the nonverbal patient can gain the nurse's attention. This maintains a connectedness even in the nurse's absence.

An attitude of nurse-caring is manifested by a soft voice, a gentle touch, completing tasks important to the patient, working unhurriedly, protecting the patient's modesty, responding with patience, alleviating pain, and giving herself and information freely. "Whatever the one-caring actually does is enhanced or diminished, made meaningful or meaningless, in the attitude conveyed to the cared-for" (Noddings, 1984, p. 64). Quinn asks, "How can I use my consciousness, my being, my voice, my touch, my face for healing" (1992, p. 27)? There is no withholding of self, information, or care.

Within an ICU, the intentional use of nursing knowledge is limited by time and other events. Yet, within a highly technical, threatening environment of an ICU, the nurse can create a healing environment by her presence, touch, voice, and manner that promotes well-being, comfort, trust, and rest. Even when the patient has lost all sense of control, the nurse can communicate that the situation is in control. Often responses will be observed in the patient's eyes. Watson (1987) believes that caring can place technology and science within the context of human meaning. To do so requires awareness and consciousness on the part of the nurse to choose a different path.

The patient, or the one-cared-for, participates in this reciprocal relationship by receiving both the nurse and the care. In this case, the patient gestured "thumbs up" to convey receiving, agreement, and approval of and to the nurse. This simple gesture confirms the nurse's actions, and he or she is in turn motivated by the knowledge that the efforts and care are received. "How good I can be is partly a function of how *you*—the other—receive and respond to me" (Noddings, 1984, p. 6). As the nurse moved between relational and analytical modes, she received positive feedback from physiologic parameters as well. For example, putting ventilated patients flat, and rolling them to give them back care or to reposition, often causes coughing, bronchospasm, or increased heart rate. The nurse is constantly processing a multitude of cues from the patient to determine the effects of his or her care. The nurse's paradigmatic perspective arranges those cues in a hierarchical order of importance.

Night 6—Crash!

I was not scheduled to work, but I was asked at 7 A.M. if I would come in for another night. I discussed this with a supervisor in front of Cathy.

I said to Cathy, "We've got a good routine here. I wouldn't mind coming in tonight and taking care of you." She smiled and gave me the thumbs up sign. So far, she had a repertoire of five hand signals. The rest of our communication was one-sided, at least verbally. I talked and she agreed or disagreed. At this point, she had monitor leads and wires, the ET tube, a nasogastric tube, a venous access device with two IV lines, the pulse oximeter on her left hand, a Foley catheter, a cold facecloth on her forehead, wet-to-dry dressings on both feet, which were up on pillows, the call bell on her belly button, and a suction catheter in her right hand.

That third night, Cathy "crashed" despite my vigilance. Her urinary output dropped, as it always did at night. I gave her some Lasix but about an hour later, she was in severe distress with dropping O_2 saturations. I motioned for the other nurse to come into the room and ordered arterial blood gases and a stat chest X-ray. I stayed with Cathy with my arms around her, speaking quietly and telling her, "You can do this."

"Do you need help?" asked the other nurse. "No, we'll be all right."

Cathy had several panic attacks on the vent but this was different. I quietly called the other nurse to get the house officer to the bedside to read the X-ray and get some morphine.

Cathy's X-ray showed a "white out," which meant fluid throughout her lungs. We changed her vent settings. "The doctor ordered 1–6 mg of morphine." She held up five fingers. "You want 5 mg?" Thumbs up. She immediately improved with the morphine.

Caring Practice: Healing, Not Curing

Caring cannot prevent untoward events. Caring from a HEC perspective can fully integrate the experience for both patient and nurse in the moment. The nurse *knew* the patient and was vigilant. But her vigilance could not prevent pulmonary edema. The nurse continued to control the environment and create a healing place with her calm appearance, voice, and touch. The nurse controlled herself and her reaction, and she consciously kept things quiet without undue alarm. She allowed the patient to choose the amount of morphine she would accept because she valued the patient as the best knower of herself as one who had lived through decades of physical illness. "I must see her as she might be—as she envisions her best self, in order to confirm her" (Noddings, 1984, p. 67). Being fully present and self-giving within an open environment allowed for energy to exchange and the experience to evolve. The humanity of the person was continually validated throughout.

Day 6—Chaos

One morning after report, Cathy had another episode of pulmonary edema. This episode was handled much differently. Cathy was sitting up gasping for air. The vent alarm was piercing. The day nurse called for help and bagged her.

"Calm down! Lay back! Relax!" they ordered her. Another nurse took over the ambu, bagged Cathy forcefully, and didn't synchronize with Cathy's own respirations. Cathy was bucking the ambu bag; the vent alarms were still screeching. The caregivers kept telling her, "Relax!" It was chaos.

"Get ABGs. Call X-ray! Get me some Lasix!" It seemed to me that Cathy was forgotten in the bed. The vent alarm was still screeching. My shift was over 30 minutes earlier. When I saw that the nurses didn't want to hear what worked before, I left the unit watching my new friend be battered—well, at least, it seemed that way to me. Awareness of the "person" was lost. My partner on nights was also aghast. Her comments were comforting to me in a strange way. I knew that she had approved of the way we handled the similar episode on nights. I couldn't change the way other nurses intervened. Yet, I trusted them completely to alleviate her symptoms—eventually.

Caring and Being Cared For

In the relational process of inclusion, the one-caring assumes a dual perspective and sees things both from the provider's own perspective and from the perspective of the one-cared-for (Noddings, 1984). Having cared for the patient for several nights in a calm, healing environment with respect for person and autonomy, and after responding to the acute episode much differently, the nurse now feels powerless. She tried to intervene, to be the patient's voice, to tell what worked before, but she was sent home.

Commentary is included as an example of the prevailing paradigmatic perspective currently present in clinical practice. Even expert nurses with decades of experience in critical care get startled with flash pulmonary edema because the patient is instantly and dramatically dyspneic. Following their paradigmatic algorithm for pulmonary edema, the day nurses focused on managing the situation, controlling the patient without regard for their inherent power as healers and creators of healing environments, unaware of the potential effects that this shift in practice may have on the patient. The nurse, in this perspective, is viewed as knower; the situation becomes what needs to be controlled, and the patient becomes objectified. The patient, fighting for every breath, is told to "lie down" and "relax" as if she had a choice in her actions. Having practiced in an ethic of caring, the nurse now experiences moral distress at the prevailing paradigm.

That's What Got Me Through

Eventually, after eight days on the vent and severe fluid restriction, Cathy was extubated and did beautifully. When I entered at 11 P.M., she put her call light on.

"I just wanted to talk to you," she said. "Thanks for all you did. Thanks for talking to me and telling me everything that was going on. Thanks for not yelling at me. Others thought I was deaf or something. Your talking to me really got me through. Once, when I was near death in a coma, Jim talked to me the whole time. That's what got me through. Talking. I'm so glad you came in that extra night!"

"Cathy, I looked at you that first night and thought, 'My God, she's my age in that bed. I'm going to treat her as I would want to be treated.' I also knew that you were the expert in your care and I needed to keep you informed."

The sweet reward in the ICU occurs when the patient, now extubated, calls the nurse into her room to tell the nurse that her care made the difference. This is a sacred moment of transformation and affirmation. The patient essentially says, "I know you were trying really hard on my behalf and what you did got me through." Isn't this nurse as healing environment? Did she call the competent but rough nurses in to say, "thanks for getting me through"?

Discussion

This chapter offers a clinical exemplar that depicts the nurse–patient dyad in the critical care setting. The dominant paradigm in the story was the particulate-deterministic perspective (Newman, Sime & Corcoran-Perry, 1991). The question to be answered was, "What is the quality of the relationship that makes it possible for the nurse and the patient to connect in a transforming way" (p. 35)?

To begin, the one-caring refused to judge but was open and receiving. The nurse did not push the patient away during their first meeting but showed openness by a soft voice, by touch, and by attending to a care routine preferred by the patient. She connected. The nurse chose not to be the authority or to exert control over the patient or her information. A sincere respect for person was shown by freely sharing vital signs, laboratory results, and doctors' orders and by allowing the patient, as expert knower of self, to choose. The nurse used her knowledge of the patient to fluidly move between relational and analytic modes but ontological knowing was valued over epistemological knowing. Even when the patient was acutely ill with pulmonary edema, the analytic mode was secondary to caring interventions. The nurse created a healing environment and incorporated the equipment as well as herself into the field. Newman describes the process as follows: "Nursing intervention is derived from a relational paradigm that directs the professional to enter into a *partnership* with the client, often at a time of chaos, with the mutual goal of participating in an authentic relationship, trusting that in the process of its unfolding, both will emerge at a higher level of consciousness" (2000, p. 97). Although the nurse in the exemplar was not working from a unitary-transformative paradigm, many of the concepts do cross into the interactive-integrative paradigm. The patient, or one-cared-for, participated in the relationship primarily through reciprocity. Her gestures, nods, postures, and facial expressions gave continuous feedback to the nurse.

As a patient–nurse dyad, however, mutuality was evident in the synchrony of care, presencing, trust, respect, and affirmation. Each partner contributed separately and mutually to produce a transforming experience. The patient was eager to speak with the nurse after extubation to tell the nurse how she "got her through." The nurse reflected on this patient by recording the experience in an exemplar. The patient was encouraged to create a journal about the experience as a way of integrating the experience (see "Aftermath"). What occurs in the patient–nurse dyad is *more than* the contributions of each person—a powerful, mutual process that changes both nurse and patient forever.

There is a need for further inquiry into the patient–nurse dyad as a transforming experience. Little in the literature addresses to the joy, happiness, or satisfaction—all powerful motivators—that nurses feel when they have given their best selves and have been received. Noddings (1984) categorizes joy as "reflective-in-nature," "a willing transformation of self" (p. 144) that "maintains us in caring" (p. 147). She likens it to the Eastern sense of oneness.

Aftermath

I visited Cathy after she left the CCU. I asked her if she kept a journal, and she said, "No." "When you get home, you may want to write about this whole thing. It's been quite an experience." Cathy was genuinely interested. I brought her an inexpensive journal. I do not know if she ever used it. I kept in touch with her for a time and found out a few years later that she had died.

Transforming Connections

This exemplar and reflection sought to answer the question posed by Newman et al.: "What is the quality of the relationship that makes it possible for the nurse and the patient to connect in a transforming way?" (1991, p. 35). The patient is ill, fearful, and vulnerable. The patient reaches out to the nurse, and the nurse physically reaches back. Through actions and words, the nurse communicates, "I am fully aware of what is happening. I hear your fear. I will respond. I understand your problem. I know how to help. I will stay with you until you tell me I can leave. I will show you how to call for help when I am not present. I will provide care in a way that gives you feelings of comfort and security. I believe you to be the best knower of yourself, and I will listen to your knowledge. I will help make this situation a good one for you. I will be watchful. I will tell you what I know and help you to interpret your environment. I will use myself and equipment to help you rest, to give you physical stability. I must continue to learn more about you so that I can promote holistic care of body, mind, and spirit." These caring operations can also be called by their conceptual names, such as presencing, reassuring, valuing, knowing, facilitating, reflecting, and vigilance. They are the key elements in the relationship that allow for transformation.

Recommendations for Education: Personal Transformation

I am often told by registered nurses who are returning to school for baccalaureate degrees, "I'm not really learning anything." From their particulate-deterministic paradigm, they may not be learning anything new in terms of nursing skills. My response is usually, "We're helping you to think differently." It is really not far from the truth. While learning new paradigmatic perspectives, nurses are encouraged to reflect upon their practice, to examine the embedded traditions in their work settings, and to "try on" new approaches. Nurses attending graduate programs often initially groan at the mention of nursing theory and look forward to the point in their studies where they can learn "useful things." Theory, learned by practicing nurses, enhances critical thinking and ethical practice. Advanced education allows nurses to bring with them vast experiences, deconstruct old traditions, and learn new paradigmatic perspectives. Good nurses become better nurses. Knowledge from multiple sources, especially nursing science, is essential for this transformation to occur.

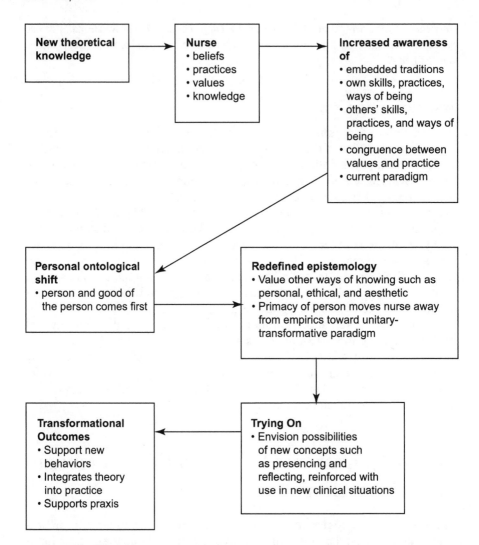

Figure 17.1.   Knowledge Synthesis: A model of nurse transformation.

The exemplar in this chapter chronicles one nurse's contextual experience. As such, it may not be generalizable. However, an inductive model is postulated in Figure 17.1. In a nursing graduate program, the nurse who had her own beliefs, practices, and values was introduced to nursing theories new to her. This led to an increased awareness in her clinical work setting, the ICU. The nurse became aware of embedded traditions and other nurses' practices, skills, and ways of being as well as her own. The nurse learned of other ways of knowing such as the ethical, aesthetic, and personal components (Chinn & Kramer, 2003) and reflected on her own practice for congruence through the questions, "Do I know what I do? Do I do what I know?"

The nurse in this story experienced an ontological shift where person superceded all other components of the metaparadigm. The good of the person came before environment, nurse, and health, with health being seen as just one aspect of the total person. The nurse redefined epistemology by discarding a priori information and no longer relied solely on empirics. Primacy of person moved the nurse away from the particulate-deterministic perspective and toward the unitary-transformative perspective.

The nurse imagined new possibilities of being; "tried on" new concepts such as presencing, reflecting, valuing, and openness; and relinquished control. The experience with this patient became a paradigm exemplar. The transforming experience, the outcome, supported the new behaviors and caused the nurse to seek similar knowledge. In this way, the theoretical knowledge was integrated with practice, not as whole theories but rather as concepts deemed congruent by the nurse.

Watson, Newman, and others have said that how we view person determines care. To progress in the twenty-first century, nurses need to question existing paradigmatic perspectives and envision outcomes under new paradigms. Nurses need to critically evaluate and deconstruct embedded traditions. Those with advanced education should model new ways of being and new ways of caring for patients in ways that reflect an ontological awareness of what it is to be human. Research is needed to provide evidence of patient outcomes under these new paradigms. Sensitive outcome measures are needed to uncover postmodern nurse–patient phenomena. Only then will we be able to answer Newman's question regarding the quality of the patient–nurse relationship, an authentic relationship where "both will emerge at a higher level of consciousness" (2000, p. 97).

References

Benner, P. (1984). *From novice to expert: Excellence and power in clinical nursing practice.* Menlo Park, CA: Addison-Wesley.

Boykin, A., & Schoenhofer, S. (1993). *Nursing as caring: A model for transforming practice.* New York, NY: National League for Nursing.

Chinn, P. L., & Kramer, M. K. (2003). *Theory and nursing: Integrated knowledge development* (6th ed.). St. Louis, MO: Mosby Year Book.

Nelms, T. P. (1996). Living a caring presence in nursing: A Heideggerian hermeneutical analysis. *Journal of Advanced Nursing*, 24, 368–374.

Newman, M. A. (1995). *A developing discipline: Selected works of Margaret Newman.* New York, NY: National League for Nursing.

Newman, M. A. (2000). *Health as expanding consciousness* (2nd ed.). New York, NY: National League for Nursing.

Newman, M. A., Sime, A., & Corcoran-Perry, S. A. (1991). The focus of the discipline of nursing. *Advances in Nursing Science*, 14(1), 1–6.

Noddings, N. (1984). *Caring: A feminine approach to ethics and moral education.* Berkeley, CA: University of California Press.

Quinn, J. (1992). Holding sacred space: The nurse as healing environment. *Holistic Nursing Practice,* 6(4), 26–36.

Radwin, L. (1996). Knowing the patient: A review of research on an emerging concept. *Journal of Advanced Nursing,* 23(6), 1142–1146.

Tanner, C., Benner, P., Chesla, C., & Gordon, D. (1993). The phenomenology of knowing the patient. *Image: Journal of Nursing Scholarship,* 25(4), 273–280.

Watson, J. (1987). Nursing on the caring edge: Metaphorical vignettes. *Advances in Nursing Science,* 10, 10–18.

PART FIVE

DIALOGUE AND COMMENTARY

CHAPTER EIGHTEEN

CONVERGENCE AND DIVERGENCE: DIALOGUE OF NURSE THEORISTS: NEWMAN, WATSON, AND ROY

CAROL PICARD

DOROTHY JONES

Introduction

During the International Association for Human Caring (IAHC) research conference in Boston in 2002, an opportunity presented itself to engage in a dialogue with three nurse leaders who have contributed much to knowledge development and nursing science overall. Present at the conference were Drs. Jean Watson and Margaret Newman, and Sr. Callista Roy. Drs. Carol Picard and Dorothy Jones met with these leaders in a private dialogue focusing on their perceptions about the future of nursing knowledge development, the potential convergence of nursing theory, and its philosophical and conceptual points of unity. This chapter presents the thinking of the group at the time of the dialogue. Also, the content of the discussion begins to uncover the links among the thinking of these leaders as well as implications for knowledge development. The Margaret Newman paper referred to in the dialogue can be found in Chapter 1 of this book.

> **Carol Picard (CP):** To begin the conversation I had shared with both of you that I had read a story by Flannery O'Connor entitled "Everything That Rises Must Converge." Dorothy and I have noticed convergence in reading your works, particularly your most recent works. Margaret, it's great to have you talk about it in your keynote address (at IAHC) where you see convergence happening. It's a real call to action for a push forward in terms of how nursing is conceptualizing knowledge, how we as a profession are conceptualizing what are our philosophy and our common values. This is

an invitation to continue the dialogue that you began. Jean, I remember at the Scotland conference of the IAHC your presentation focused on similar dimensions. This meeting is time to begin just that, to think about this convergence.

Jean Watson (JW): Well, I thought Margaret's paper was really pace setting and exciting for me to feel like this International Caring Conference was actually starting to clarify the discipline for the next millennium or this millennium, and the future in bringing some of the work on caring together. Expanding consciousness was really a beautiful contribution of all of us—a special gift intellectually and otherwise. I think we've all been kind of isolated in the silos of nursing theory—all these separate things to see ultimately there is convergence. You really take it to a higher order or deeper order. And for me, I guess, putting caring into the model not only is congruent with what you unraveled for us and began to reflect to us and integrate, but is also a moral foundation of the profession, which I think is really very important to have as the value of foundation. Once you put caring into the framework, you automatically have a relational kind of model, and it's an ethical kind of moral position for the profession. I think that's another piece that can be acknowledged.

Margaret Newman (MN): Yes, it was kind of a surprise for me to see how many people are putting it together. When I started looking at some of the other literature and saw these terms that combine caring and knowing, I think there's real hope.

JW: What I liked about your model was that other term, "consciousness." It manifests more love and ultimately the infinity of the higher consciousness. It is really a manifestation of love and then you're into infinity and into spirit. And it opens up lots of things.

CP: In 1997, I remember the tenth anniversary issue of *Nursing Science Quarterly*. You each did a piece on where we are now, and I think that might have been the issue where Callista also expanded her philosophical assumptions in the direction we're talking about. Now the point is, for me, when I think about convergence happening—I can see it happening in your respective writings.

MN: I felt that way about Callista's work. I heard her present it at the Boston Knowledge Development Conference and thought (inwardly smiling), "sounds like expanding consciousness to me."

Dorothy Jones (DJ): Do you think, though, as you're talking, that every theorist would agree caring is manifested in each respective theory? It would give caring a different kind of universal perspective on the nature of the discipline for that particular theorist to interpret. Or is it, for example, like Margaret's discussion of caring in relation to her thinking, Jean's discussion of caring in relation to her thinking? Is caring the universal core? Is it a universal construct that filters through all or is there some type of convergence between a caring philosophy and these other theoretical positions? Do you have any thoughts about it?

JW: I'm saying if you have caring—I mean once you put caring into the disciplinary matrix, it is a universal piece and the reason I say it's universal is because of the ethical piece. And more recently, one of the things I've been into (of course, I'm going in all kinds of directions right now) is that I've been reading more and more of Levinas' work. He's a French philosopher. He talks about ethics as the first principle—the ethics of faith, this relational piece that is actually critiquing Heidegger and beyond just the ontology of care which leads into the relational ontology. But the notion of caring as first principle is the ethical foundation; you can't get away from that relationship piece. Then it gets into pattern between the spin-off and the two. Caring is the ethical core for the discipline and for the professional practice. People could come at it from whatever lens they wish to use to reflect their theoretical perspective. I think this is happening with this evolution of even what Margaret was presenting yesterday [see Chapter 1]. It's almost as if it's clarifying the disciplinary matrix in a way that then you can have multiple theories once you have this kind of solidifying—I don't want to say "solidifying" in a set way, but in a more consolidating way or an integrating way. Then it gives the big picture. And then you can have multiple things happening within it. As you say, it transcends, it accommodates anything that comes before it. So that is my way of maybe thinking about that.

DJ: But it seems like caring as a universal core around which you can get the greatest conceptual consensus.

CP: Except it's not a consensus—okay, let's hear about that.

MN: For nursing we have to have something beyond caring. It has to be conditional, so to speak, in terms of our arena of practice. As far as I'm concerned, our arena of practice is focused on health, and there are a lot of different kinds of health. There could be caring in relation to a medical model of health or some other model of health, as well as health as expanding consciousness. We can't just stop at caring.

JW: That's why I have increasingly started linking caring and healing to make this connection, because it can't be just caring by itself. It's really caring in the human health/illness–healing experience, with health even the human experience regardless . . . it's about the human and that's what nursing does within that relationship. It transcends any kind of health/illness condition.

MN: Martha [Rogers] centered on the human being, and she never elaborated what health is—or caring. She didn't see caring as being unique to nursing and, therefore, did not see it as the focus of the discipline. It is an evolutionary kind of thing in terms of the way the concepts come together.

JW: And I don't think she ever really ever understood caring as the way in which I've actually tried to describe it. It is an epistemic as well as an ethical perspective. It's not just caring as a little nice, kind way to be—it's not that kind of nursing. It's the epistemology, the ontology.

MN: But this is part of the evolution of things because the early theorists (I mean the people who were called "theorists"; there are a lot of people who are theorists who are not called theorists) found it hard to come together around caring. I take myself out of that a little bit, to look beyond what was developed in the early stages of nursing theory.

DJ: I think of you all as pioneers. It was a wave of knowledge development that was silo driven, true, but absolutely necessary that there be a generation to take the discipline forward in a way that really hadn't happened prior. I would imagine that as you are developing your own work it is pretty energy intensive, and you do stay focused to take your own work forward. But something is happening with this idea of convergence, a blending of perspectives. What's different?

MN: I hear a lot of feedback from students who are not bound by those previous perspectives. As hard as it is to hear something outside your own silo, so to speak, you have to listen because these are bright individuals who are very committed to nursing and committed to nursing knowledge and they're saying something a little bit different. So you have to open your eyes to that, and I'm just so pleased that we're at this point.

JW: It's refreshing. It's liberating because we have been shut down and I just really have thought it was destructive to the profession and to nursing knowledge development to have these categories set. It's like Levinas, who talks about totalizing something or the infinity versus totality, and it's like we're totalizing a theory by setting it in *this* category and setting it in *this* core paradigm and forever stuck in critiquing it. On the one hand, okay, it helps to see these different things; on the other hand, it sets the ideas and prevents the evolution of nursing. Now it's loosening up, and there are multiple paradigms. Or the paradigm itself is expanded in a way that it can accommodate multiple perspectives on various phenomena.

DJ: It seems like as a science is growing and the knowledge of the science is developing, people are more cognizant of grounding their work, and often found grounding in other sciences. If you look at psychiatry, for example, it has multiple perspectives that directly relate to the way care is given—how treatment is planned. Do you see maybe the growth of nursing—the evolution of the practice, the growth of knowledge—coming together?

MN: People are searching. I don't want my work to be seen as coming out of another discipline. I see it as emerging from a nursing paradigm.

CP: Welcome, Callista. I started our conversation by saying that there's a short story by Flannery O'Connor entitled "Everything That Rises Must Converge," and we had a really wonderful keynote paper from Margaret, who was speaking to that as part of her presentation. We were just talking about convergence and about how that may be the next level or next wave of development in the discipline. We're very interested to hear about your thoughts on that. Jean also had responded to some of the things that Margaret had said around the whole notion of caring, and Margaret introduced more of that concept in her presentation. We were looking at the distinction of caring.

JW: It could also be somewhat of a spin-off of some of the work that Marlaine Smith and I did two years ago on the Rogerian and caring science model; this became a more specific kind of focus on that. As I have read and seen your [Callista Roy's] more recent works in the last five years or so, it's just incredible now hearing the whole cosmology as well. It's like something is happening in the universe.

Callista Roy (CR): I actually started this in 1983, and I agree. I think the whole idea of convergence and the higher levels of unity are manifesting in many, many different ways. Interestingly enough, what I heard on public radio coming down to this meeting was a focus on literature and medicine by physicians who write poetry. I think we were on the right track all the way along from Florence Nightingale, but it is just a terribly exciting time for knowledge. I think about the incredible science and philosophy of the twentieth century, and then just taking that leap into the twenty-first century will give us all kinds of possibilities. There are so many people who have written in science, who then end up with very philosophical sorts of analysis of conscilience. The other fellow I think of is Ken Wilber, a developmental psychologist, who wrote about the eye of the spirit or an integral vision. I think it is definitely the case that in general there are more and more ways in which knowledge and world perspectives perhaps are converging and using many different ways of getting at knowledge—ways of knowing. I would also agree with that about our work.

For myself, not only do I have all kinds of influences on myself personally, but I also think the influences are different—writing, reading, listening here, talking . . . In some cases for me, it's also been hearing an idea and saying, "No, I'm thinking of something a little bit different," so I've got to then figure out how to articulate it. That's where the first stimulus came at the Rogers conference in 1983. I'd been feeling this for a long time. I felt there is a difference here, and is it a questioned, regional difference: East versus West? I went to the 1983 conference to learn more about what was going on and what Rogers was saying and to hear the other papers. I was walking across Times Square to meet somebody for dinner and I thought, "You know, there's just something more to it. What is that?" The next morning one of the first papers talked about relativity as a primary assumption of Rogers' book. That is not my belief; therefore, what is it? So that's where I started on this track. I had an invitation to speak at the University of San Francisco, a Jesuit institution, as a clinical nurse scholar because I was a post-doc at the time at the University of California at San Francisco. They were opening a whole discussion on ethics and science, and this was the kickoff presentation. Speaking can crystallize ideas. The whole line of questioning at that Rogerian meeting gave me the urge to do something. I started articulating it first in one speech. From there, the next major link would have been to the 1988 paper with an explication of the philosophical assumptions of the Roy model in the first issue of Nursing *Science Quarterly*. I was asked to write some things. Then 10 years later, they asked me to do a retrospective. By then, I was in Boston, teaching and writing with nurses. In addition, I belong to an interdisciplinary group called "the faith and science exchange" of the Boston Theological Institute. It is a wonderful group of scholars, including astronomers, chemists, and others of Islamic, Jewish, and Christian traditions who are a huge influence on me. This is just one example of influences I have in my life all the time. The other thing is my personal spiritual life, where I have encountered brilliant thinkers in earth-based spirituality such as Thomas Berry. Those are some of the personal influences on me, so at the same time I'm reading and listening as I think and write. The Nursing Knowledge Conference series here in New England has also had an influence on me. I wrote a paper on knowledge as universal cosmic imperative. From there, I've been working with some of the ideas of purposefulness. What do I mean by that? I am further into the philosophical assumption of veritivity and then the implications of that.

Some of the international work—in particular, Eastern thinking—has also influenced me. I've had a visitor come for a short post-doc experience. She wanted to talk to me about some of my philosophical assumptions related to the Asian cultures. I thought, "I'm not going to do this alone," so I got a small group to join me: a graduate of the Boston College Ph.D. in nursing program from mainland China, a colleague from Korea, a current doctoral student from Thailand, and a recent Ph.D. graduate who has done a lot of work with veritivity and has actually developed an instrument. The group joined me to engage in this dialogue. So my thinking is truly influenced by this kind of cross-fertilizing dialogue.

DJ: We were talking before about just getting into the discussion about the substantive content of the discipline. Are we any closer to bringing forth consistently the content that really defines and refines nursing? We have consistency around nursing process maybe, but this discussion is introducing us into a whole new direction. Is there any consensus around bringing this perspective forward so that nursing can better articulate its science? Further, can we set an educational standard that defines essential knowledge as part of the curriculum? Research obviously helps us build that, but we lack consistency, which then, I think, compromises nursing's potential.

CP: What I've seen happen in both undergraduate and graduate programs is that theory is not lived out in explicating practice. It is compartmentalized as content and not lived through a curriculum. Programs teach about disease and not the whole. We are unclear about our purpose.

JW: There's only one master's practitioner program that requires theory by practice. That is the American Holistic Nurses Association practitioner program. It is the only certification for advanced practice that absolutely requires the practice be grounded in nursing theory. All the others are basically atheoretical. They might study it, but it's not something that guides their practice intentionally. One of the questions I have—and it's probably not answering Dorothy's question, but it's something that I'm struggling with—is about this spiraling in this convergence and the connections. When you move to kind of a unitary perspective and make nursing more explicit, you get into energy and you get into spirit. What I want to acknowledge is that it is experiential. You really have to honor your working with the light.

MN: I agree that it is experiential. That's the reason I have shifted from calling our knowledge "science" and now refer to it as "praxis," the merging of theory, research, and practice. The literature supports the synthesis of caring and health with the underlying concepts of wholeness, pattern, mutual process, consciousness, transcendence, and transformation. The following statement, which I quote from my recent article in *Advances in Nursing Science* [vol. 26, no. 4, pp. 240–245, 2003], was compiled from authors representing a variety of theoretical persuasions [refer to the article for the sources of the statements] and illustrates the convergence of our thinking:

> The nursing mandate is to address the wholeness of the human being through caring, including a notion of health that spans all dimensions of life. Health incorporates wellness, illness, well-being, and disease into a larger whole. In the discipline statement, "caring in the human health experience," caring and health can be seen as dialectically related . . . they merge as the process of expanding consciousness. Wholeness is the starting point with caring as the moral ideal. Healing is not seeking a desired wholeness but rather is realizing an inherent wholeness. Healing is the process of realizing one's pattern (wholeness). Pattern is central

to nursing; the theories of nursing focus on life's meanings. Meaning and consciousness are constitutive of person–environment integration . . . life has transcendent meaning. Transformation comes about in the process of pattern recognition through the dialectics of theory in action. Nursing as mutual process is evidenced in dialogue, which is the interpenetrability of consciousness and uniqueness of meaning in nurse–patient encounters. Nursing connects with deeply felt experience and meaning, has the capacity to step into another reality, to shift experience into a different realm. There is a connection between self-transcendence and personal transformation relevant to expanding consciousness. Consciousness is information in the form of pattern and meaning; expanding consciousness is seen in deepening meaning, insight, new ways of relating to self and other. (p. 243)

CR: I find more interest in theory-based practice in my experiences around the United States and in other countries than Jean notes. I do agree with some of Margaret's identified points of convergence—notably, nursing knowledge and practice focused on wholeness, pattern, mutual life processes, consciousness, transcendence, and transformation. One particular point of divergence that I think remains in our literature is our ambivalence about relativism, particularly as influenced by postmodern thinking. That is why I will continue to articulate the common purposefulness of humankind, cosmic unity, and what I call veritivity.

CP/DJ: Thank you for the opportunity to talk together and reflect on the state of nursing science and knowledge development. It has been a unique and historical dialogue.

Chapter Nineteen

Dialogue of Newman Scholars and Others Interested in HEC

Katherine Rosa

Introduction

In May 2002, nurses interested in discussing nursing science from a unitary-transformative perspective and, in particular, the theory of health as expanding consciousness (HEC) met in Boston. This meeting followed the twenty-fourth annual conference of the International Association for Human Caring (IAHC), where many of those gathered had presented papers and workshops. The group included clinicians, educators, and researchers from across the United States, Canada, England, Iceland, New Zealand, and Australia. The dialogue that ensued offered participants an opportunity to discuss HEC from multiple perspectives.

Among those present at this meeting was Dr. Margaret Newman. Many of the group participants embodied the theory of HEC within their clinical practice, teaching, and research programs so there were many shared beliefs in the group. The dialogue emerged within an environment of care in which the discussion was respectful, reflective, and fluid in movement. Throughout the dialogue, Dr. Newman gently reminded participants to let go of mental barriers that could block the unfolding of pattern. Thus the meeting was one of praxis, in which experiences were shared, theory reflected upon, meanings postulated, and new options explored. This chapter highlights some of the themes that emerged from the dialogue. It includes the structure and process changes that occur when using HEC in nursing practice and education, nursing science and art, and nursing knowledge, philosophy, presence, and intentionality.

HEC: Nursing Education and Practice

The group participants agreed that HEC-based nursing was foundationally different from traditional nursing observed within the discipline. The structure and process of traditional nursing education and clinical practice often gave limited attention to nursing theory as subject matter and even less attention to its application in practice. In opposition to this perspective, HEC is viewed as process, an embodied invitation by the nurse to intentionally promote a patient/client/family partnership and reflect on personal meaning and choice within a relationship at times of profound vulnerability.

Professor Dawn Freshwater, from Bournemouth University in England, expressed her concern that student nurses were often encouraged to look mainly to the literature for knowledge as evidence about practice, without some measure of attention being paid to their own direct experience with the person. Freshwater has found that students are rarely asked to express their own wisdom gained through an experience during their clinical descriptions of care. If the important evidence of relationship is discounted, their developing presence with the patient is devalued, and the awareness of the unfolding of meaning within the nurse–patient relationship is lost. The richness and potential of the relationship becomes secondary to a problem-oriented interventionist approach. Freshwater suggested a narrative approach to teaching HEC, by inviting the students to tell their own stories about an encounter.

Dr. Fran Reeder, a nursing professor at the University of Colorado, suggested that faculty need to teach theory to graduate students in a way congruent with practice. According to her, graduate students have been demoralized and mired in the medical model. Teaching theory to graduate students provides them with a language to understand the process of personal unfolding. As educators nurture the individual's sense of self, students can make the connection to increased awareness within their clinical experiences and discuss patients' experiences from a perspective other than medicine.

Many of those present agreed that demands of the practice setting and the speed with which patients and information processing need to occur have promoted a skill-oriented, competency-based, *doing for* the patient and family rather than *being with* and journeying with the patients and families as they cope with illness or promote health. One participant noted how hard it was to *be with* the patient. She discussed the art of balance was critical to achieving this goal. Margaret Newman advised the group to be fully present with the patient and family, trust the process as the essence of praxis, and remember that the process was evolving for teacher and learner.

Dr. Dorothy Jones invited those gathered to imagine how HEC scholars, teachers, and clinicians could move a HEC-based praxis approach along when powerful dichotomies persist within practice models and curricula. She asked the group to consider the moral challenges associated with nurse educators who exposed students to ideal patient care experiences guided by theory such as HEC, only to have the demands of the practice setting force the learner into a more technically driven practice. Some consensus was reached that the moral obligation was to teach the science and work to change practice environments, now.

Dr. Carolyn Hayes, a nurse researcher and clinician as well as nurse ethicist, suggested that it was important to pay attention to nurses already engaged in practice. She pointed out that there are opportunities to make incremental changes in the practice environment and nurses are eager to practice within a nursing framework. Sue Hagedorn, a Colorado-based nurse practitioner and educator, observed that even during short appointments with patients, it was possible to purposefully attend to meaning and pattern with people. In her practice, she worked to create "sacred space" in each clinical encounter. Another nurse wondered how to maintain this sensibility: "There is not support in the environment. It is very isolating in practice." The group agreed that it was important to talk with scholars who could be supportive and encourage a nursing-focused practice.

Merian Litchfield, a HEC scholar and nurse consultant from New Zealand, suggested that it was important for the group members to view nursing as separate from organizational structures. Her vision was to expand the dialogue beyond a personal framework of nursing practice to the creation of a new model for practice. Some participants supported this perspective, saying that it was impossible for nurses to practice in two different paradigms and that it was time to stop trying. Dr. Jane Flanagan, nurse clinician and researcher, shared that nurse participants in her research noted the value of focusing on patients from a HEC perspective. Findings from her study suggested that staff found that the process affirmed the reason why they became nurses in the first place. It was the art of nursing lived fully in relationship that nurses using a HEC framework experienced. Many said they could "never go back" to their old practice orientation. This perspective helped to change a system of care within one practice setting and increased patient and nurse satisfaction overall.

Nursing Knowledge and Art

At the IAHC conference, one keynote presenter was an artist who spoke about the role of art with people who are ill. During her experiences with patients, it was important to stay open to those with whom she collaborated, and to create art that reflected personal life meanings. The dialogue explored the nature of art and nursing knowledge. Was there philosophically a difference between nurses and this artist? What was it the role of both as providers of care? The consensus of the group was that the difference lay in the goals of each discipline. The goal of nursing was to promote healing. Art could be viewed as a strategy to achieve this goal. For the artist, art was the creation of something that had meaning and was a source of joy, beauty, or mystery depending on perceptions of all present. The focus of the artist is in the art. The nurse uses art to uncover human expression within the life story. Yet, a question soon surfaced; "Is the theory of HEC broader than the discipline?" This query generated a general discussion that led to some agreement that the process itself takes place within the discipline, with an awareness that HEC has implications beyond the discipline.

Nursing Knowledge, Philosophy, Intentionality, and Presence

Some attendees at the meeting also practiced within Watson's "theory of caring" framework, in which intentionality for healing is an element of caring practice. These participants questioned the similarity between Watson's caring theory and HEC-based practice. Sue Hagedorn shared that she used intention to create a caring environment by embracing the moment and making it her intention to be of help. Others spoke of the need to create a "sacred space" through intention; if one sits in presence and hopes for presence, they noted, then that is what one intends. Another participant cited Husserl, noting that intentionality is a human capacity. Inherent in our perceiving something, judging something, willing something, enjoying something, and hoping for something is the notion that movement toward something evolves out of the relational encounter. The distinction between intention and intentionality was examined through participants' personal experiences.

One person cautioned that there seemed to be an outcome-oriented approach to intentionality. A few scholars suggested that when intention was linked to a specific goal, it could create a restrictive boundary. For example, one person thought that if a faculty member has the intention of students' transformation, it might create a barrier to the way students' patterns unfold. The dialogue continued, linking intentionality to the being-ness of one person toward another, a focus on being present in the moment, and openness to whatever presents itself. Sitting with this tension, Merian Litchfield commented, "I can't see how nurses shift from one paradigm to another—being with and doing for . . . . The main struggle is to have it together in your mind. We are talking about an embodiment of theory. The intention is to be unintentional." There was also discussion on the similarities and differences between HEC and Watson's theory of caring.

Author's Reflection

While writing this chapter, I thought: Is the intention to create a caring environment a "doing for" rather than "being with"? Had I shifted from doing for an individual to doing for the environment in service of the individual (nurse and patient/family)? If yes, then is this shift a pattern for me? If, as the dialogue suggested, I'm not alone in my wondering, does this represent a shift in pattern manifestation of HEC nursing's evolving nature? Or, in fact, is paying greater attention to the environment the obvious next step to accelerate transformation for all involved in the partnership? I realized that the use of intentionality was connected to descriptions such as wholeness, being-ness, and openness. It is presence, in addition to personal meaning, value, and perceptions, that moves the process of HEC. A caring encounter naturally evolves from this heart-to-heart connection. And so I ask, does this mean nursing is consciously evolving toward "being for" and "doing with"?

Closing

As the meeting came to an end, one person suggested that for HEC-based practice to become mainstream, its practitioners must expand their visibility and commitment to nursing knowledge. Another participant commented that we need to remain open to the unfolding process that may move the theory/praxis of HEC forward.

As the dialogue drew to a close, Margaret Newman was asked to reflect on the dialogue. She commented that she believed the most important thing nurses could do is to trust the process of consciousness unfolding. According to Newman, an organized approach is not needed to move the theory of HEC into mainstream nursing; instead, nurses need to live the theory and its effect will spread. She said, "You catch it like you catch the flu." Participation in dialogue such as this group offers one way to create a shift in consciousness within the discipline.

Readers are referred to *www.healthasexpandingconsciousness.org* for the opportunity to converse with others interested in HEC and to find publications related to the theory.

Participants in the Dialogue

Linda Andrist, Ann-Marie Barron, Christine Bridges, Patrick Dean, John Deckro, Sharon Falkenstern, Jane Flanagan, Dawn Freshwater, Sue Hagedorn, Carolyn Hayes, Alex Hoyt, Dorothy Jones, Merian Litchfield, Arlene Lowenstein, Margaret Newman, Maggie Dexheimer Pharris, Carol Picard , Elizabeth Predeger, Fran Reeder, Katherine Rosa, Sandra Ruka, Susan Ruka, Kathleen Solomon, Katherine Lizzie Teichler, Lynne Wagner, Barbara Zust.

Chapter Twenty

The Impact of HEC: Concluding Thoughts and Future Directions

Dorothy A. Jones

The discussions, reflections, and insights presented throughout this text support Newman's (1994) theoretical assumptions underlying health as expanding consciousness (HEC). This theoretical perspective provides a guide to research as praxis, innovation in clinical practice, and curriculum development and implementation across specialties settings and groups. HEC speaks to the basic ontology of nursing, the relationship between the nurse and the patient. Within this partnership lie opportunities for discovery, awareness, choice, and transformation through a process dialogue between the patient (family and community) as well as with the nurse.

The opportunity to give voice to what nurses come to know about the human experience through purposeful, intentional presence with the patient and his or her environment is realized through HEC. Once exposed to the potential of HEC praxis, nurses find it difficult to see their care as task-oriented and recognize once again those fundamental values and beliefs that drew them to nursing. Students exposed to learning experiences guided by HEC recognize nursing's unique opportunity to be part of patients' "sacred space" in times of health and illness. This realization gives new meaning to encounters with patients and highlights nursing's unique contribution to patient care.

Knowledge within HEC can also be used to reshape clinical practice, create innovative practice models, and develop a caring environment that fosters renewal and healing for provider and patient. Practicing within such an environment offers multiple opportunities to come to know patients and their experiences in a new way, and to use research from within the nurse–patient partnership to study pattern appraisal and pattern reflection as a strategy for initiating life changes and transitions that are transformational.

Theory, Practice, Research: An Iterative Process

Theory, research, and practice are iterative and relate to one another in a "reciprocal, cyclical and interactive way" (McEwen & Willis, 2002, p. 80). Theory is tested and validated through research. Findings from research are used to refine the theory and further validate through continuous research. As the theory becomes more stable, it can be used to guide clinical practice and inform the role of nursing practice.

The clinical practice environment acts as a stimulus for inquiry. It is the laboratory of the nurse scientist, the environment in which the human experience can be understood through process. Some nurse researchers reflect on a particular experience or clinical situations and discuss phenomena related to an event. Other nurses use dialogue and narration to inquire about an experience from the patient's perceptions—i.e., "Tell me about the people and events that give your life meaning." When guided by a theoretical framework such as HEC, the lens on the nurse–client partnership is individualized, and the unique moment created jointly by the nurse and the patient becomes the setting for personal discovery, reflection, and expanding consciousness. Research provides the nurse with knowledge about the human experience.

Theory and HEC

For Newman, health is expanding consciousness. HEC is grounded in the following assumptions:

- Health is a unitary process of the whole.
- Disease and nondisease are expressions of the whole.
- Pattern is the evolving human/environment process characterized by meaning.
- Consciousness is the informational capacity of the whole revealed in the evolving pattern of the whole. (Newman, 1994, 2002)

The theory is supported by the thinking of other scientists:

- Rogers: perspective on unitary, irreducible humans, their environment, and evolving pattern (1970).
- Young: individual movement through stages of consciousness toward ultimate freedom by recognizing choice and establishing "new rules" (1976)

- Prigogine: theory of dissipative structures; the impact of disruptive events leading to periods of disorganization and uncertainty followed by emergence of a new order and higher organization (1976)
- Bentov: description of consciousness as the informational capacity of a system viewed through the way the system interacts with the environment (1978)
- Bohm: discussion of the way implicate order is revealed through the external manifestations of the explicate order to synthesize disease as a manifestation of health (1980)

HEC proposes a shift in thinking to articulate the uniqueness of the nursing discipline as opposed to describing nursing as a role or related functions. This shift focuses on engagement between the nurse and the patient in partnership within an environment of care that moves nursing from treatment of symptoms and doing for the patient to a process in search of meaning and pattern. Within this perspective, illness is not viewed as a negative experience but rather one that can facilitate self-growth, allow reorganization, and lead to higher consciousness (Newman, 1994).

Dudley-Brown (1997, p. 101) offers several criteria with which to evaluate a theory. Newman's HEC appears to meet those criteria, consistently. The theory *accurately* describes nursing. This is influenced by the willingness of nurses across a variety of settings to embrace HEC philosophically. It appears that Newman's theoretical position is reflective of essential values and beliefs of the discipline. However, this thinking can be compromised in healthcare environments that are product driven and fast paced or when academic settings are skills oriented and disease driven to the exclusion of disciplinary knowledge.

The theory is *consistent* in that it is logical, with the definitions of terms, concepts, and statements addressed in a similar way throughout the theory. As evidenced by the many authors who have embraced the work of Newman in research and practice, the theory is also *fruitful*. HEC has been used in a variety of settings and across cultures. Results have yielded new information about humans and life experiences in health and illness.

The theory is *simple* and *complex* at the same time. The invitation to engage in the dialogue is driven by the intentional presence and purposefulness of the nurse to engage in a process with the person (or family or community) through dialogue that focuses on life meaning. The theory becomes complex when the client reflects on pattern, recognizes choices, and sees the support and knowledge needed to change. The model is broad in its *scope*, embracing multiple dimensions of practice, and is *accepted* by others in the nursing community as an important nursing theory (Chinn & Kramer, 1999; McEwen & Willis, 2002, p. 102). As evidenced in the preceding chapters, the theory has broad social utility. It is used across administrative, practice, and educational settings and is relevant to the values and beliefs of many different cultures.

Research and HEC

Knowledge developed using HEC as a framework for research has been found to uncover information that helps illuminate the meaning of the person's present situation within the context of the past and anticipating future action, and stimulates new insights that lead to clarity of action. "The hermeneutic dialectic method is used to allow the pattern of person and environment to reveal itself without disturbing the unity of the pattern. The process culminates in intuitive apprehension and expression" (Newman, 2002). The research process focuses on the following aspects:

- Creation of an environment to allow a mutual process of inquiry to occur
- Engagement in dialogue that focuses on meaningful life events and relationships for the participants
- Organization of narrative data and development of a graphic display that organizes the portrayal of the narrative in evolving patterns (e.g., developmental) over time
- Sharing of the researcher's perceptions of pattern obtained through the dialogue process with the participant for accuracy, reflection, and expansion
- Valuing the opportunity for participants to gain insights through pattern recognition that can illuminate action possibilities (Newman, 1994)

Research as praxis is defined as "thoughtful reflection and action that occur in synchrony, in the direction of transforming the world" (Wheeler & Chinn, 1984, p. 2). For praxis to occur, "not only must it illuminate the lived experience . . . it must also be illuminated by their struggles." For Newman, the "research must focus on the reality of practice" (1994, p. 92). Research emanating from the nurse's engagement with the participant on the events and relationships important to the individual's life experience enables pattern recognition and expanding consciousness to occur. "The process of nursing practice is the content of nursing research" (Newman, 1994, p. 92).

Presentations included in this text have addressed the use of research as praxis. Through pattern recognition, participants have described a new awareness about life events, relationships, and choices. Using HEC as praxis, researchers described participants who found the process illuminating, and within the process found meaning and freedom to engage even in a peaceful death (Barron, 2000). Other studies described participants who recognized the impact of life events on the present and became aware of the importance of "letting go" or "accepting" past life events so that they could move forward with their life choices (Picard, 2000). Several authors reported the importance of sustained support during periods of disruption and turbulence as essential to transformation and expanding consciousness (Berry, 2002). Pattern analysis and pattern display suggests that when support of any kind is not present, participants can get "stuck" and be unable to move on in their lives. Traumatic and disruptive events in childhood were also recognized as interfering with pattern evolution (Novolesky-Rosenthal, 1996; Capasso, 2000). This was often manifested by interruptions in communication and disconnections with significant family relationships. Pattern recognition in patients with ovarian cancer (Endo, 2000) and rheumatoid arthritis (Neill, 2002) helped to focus actions that enhanced life choices. Work with prisoners (Pharris, 2002) and families coping with a chronic illness (Picard & Margolis, 2002) described how disruptions in patterns for individuals can result in changes for families as a whole.

For many, the illness experience was seen as an opportunity for growth and change. Pattern within HEC is defined as "relatedness . . . characterized by movement diversity and rhythm" (McEwen & Willis, 2002, p. 190). Time and space may be reflected as temporal patterns or as a way of being in the world. Pattern reflection offered participants an opportunity to recognize the truth of the lived experience, find meaning, illuminate struggles in a new way, and use the illness experience to seek new opportunities for life changes.

Using research as praxis offers the researcher who embodies the theory HEC to come to a new understanding about the human experience in its totality. Illness becomes a manifestation of the whole, a way for the humanity of the person–environment experience to be revealed. Insights gained through the process affect both the nurse and the patient. This mutual process of engagement establishes a connection with the provider that is authentic. The participant comes to trust the process, and the outcome has meaning that is personal, unfolding, and open to new awareness and expanded consciousness. Changes in physical health status may provide additional manifestation of holistic healing (Capasso, 2000).

Application: Practice and Education

The use of HEC in practice and education is essential. A reciprocal relationship exists between both elements. For nurses to practice within the HEC framework, they must be exposed to the knowledge embedded in the theory and see it operationalized in learning experiences throughout a curriculum. Clinical experiences, purposefully developed to link theory and practice, can promote learning, increase sensitivity to the patient experience, and foster the student's sense of self as a nurse (Novolesky-Rosenthal & Solomon, 2001).

In addition, supportive nursing leadership within a healthcare setting and commitment to innovation in patient care can optimize the impact of theory—in particular, HEC—within practice. Developing staff and creating the dialogue with clinicians as discussed by Coakley and Coakley (Chapter 10) can be a stimulus for change. The freedom experienced by providers who are able to discuss challenges of practice along with supportive environments for exploring new directions can prove motivating for the nurse. The process gives the nurse permission for "out of the box" thinking and innovation in care delivery practices.

The new practice environments guided by HEC can be life changing for patients and staff. When HEC was actualized in a preadmission testing area (PATA), it brought new meaning and insights for the patient and the nurse (Flanagan, Chapter 5). Additional interventions, such as meditation and therapeutic touch, not only relaxed the patients but also fostered meaningful dialogue between the nurse and the patient not just in PATA but on the units as well. Patients often returned to talk with the nurses in PATA to say that their hospital experience "changed their lives."

Ruka (2003) also worked with staff in a nursing home to change the patient care delivery model for individuals experiencing Alzheimer's disease. Within this HEC-guided practice model, families were invited to share their stories about the patient. This knowledge was used to increase the nurse's knowledge about the patient and helped to guide the development of creative interventions to promote calm and healing, especially when patients expressed resistive behaviors. While the shift was important to staff, families were also able to share "their stories" and were comforted by the experience.

HEC: Future Directions

> It is time for
> A parting with the past
> It is time to
> Replace the anchor of the past
> With the pull of the future
>
> (Newman, 1994, p. 137)

Today more than ever, society needs nursing. Nursing, as a discipline, values health and the human experience in a unique way. Preserving the intrinsic dignity and worth of person (family and community) is a central focus of nursing. This discipline seeks to address the human experience in its totality. The connection created within the nurse–patient relationship fosters trust and personal discovery. Through this dialogue, patients uncover meaning and come to know the experience and understand meaning. Nursing care is an intentional, authentic, spiritual, purposeful experience with individuals that reflects the values and beliefs of the discipline and focuses on the presence of the nurse to use knowledge and promote healing (Jones, 2001).

HEC: Future Considerations

As noted in the *Consensus Document*, "nursing theory expresses the values and beliefs of the discipline, helps to frame the human experience and guides the caring process" (1998, p. 4). HEC is a stable, theoretically sound, and useful grand theory designed to offer clinicians, researchers, educators, and administrators a way to articulate the discipline and guide its essential focus: the partnership between nurse and patient. The theory is true to its underlying assumptions and, when subjected to testing through research, generates new knowledge for the discipline. Recently, there has been more attention paid to theoretical convergence as discussed by the theorists in Chapter 19. Here we focus on some future considerations for the use and development of the HEC theory.

Research as Praxis

- Continue the focus on research emanating from the practice. Expand the use of HEC with populations having more diverse cultural and ethnic backgrounds. In addition, increased attention to the use of the model with children and expanded use with families and communities are essential.
- Within the research methodology, researchers have an opportunity to reflect on the dialogue with the client at least twice. Some researchers have suggested this contact may need to increase. There is a need to consider longitudinal studies to evaluate changes over time. A time rationale for pattern reflection should be reviewed in light of new research findings. Physical indicators may be considered a manifestation of movement, personal transformation, and holistic healing.
- Continue to explore complimentary pattern recognition with use of aesthetic expression such as art, dance, or personal drawings to reflect the pattern of the whole (Picard, 2000) to understand the meaning.
- Newman considers the hermeneutic dialectic method of inquiry to be a useful methodology in uncovering pattern. The focus is on the individual. Questions have been raised about the use of this method to look across participants' patterns and the use of multiple method approaches for theme identification. Newman believes that the emphasis must be placed on the client pattern, as this is where practice lies. Continued dialogue may be needed to clarify HEC as a phenomenology (process) and as a method of inquiry. (Newman, TETRA on-line dialogue among scholars.)
- Using HEC as a research method of inquiry can guide the development of a program of research. Some researchers have gone on to expand a research program using quantitative and other qualitative research methodologies. There is a tension between HEC and traditional methods that needs further discussion.

Clinical Practice and Innovation

- Pattern appraisal and pattern recognition are useful strategies to differentiate nursing practice from other disciplines.

- Findings from pattern recognition reflection and resulting action on the part of the nurse and participant need to be communicated and studied in relation to organizational goals such as early discharge and decreased recidivism and healing. This may require redefining evidence-based practice within the HEC framework.
- Guidelines for the creation of theory-based practice models (especially HEC) need to be developed to help clinicians implement and sustain modes of care guided by HEC.
- Nursing administrators considering implementation of new practice models should consider HEC as a framework and monitor its effects on variables such as patient/family satisfaction, nurse satisfaction and professional growth, achievement of organizational goals, and cost savings.

Education

- Overall, increased attention to the goals of nursing science and the impact of nursing knowledge needs to be addressed throughout the curriculum, not just in one course. The value of nursing knowledge and theory is reflected in the curriculum and clinical experiences.
- Creative learning experiences using theory such as HEC should be studied and reported in the literature. Use of HEC in teaching and learning encounters changes the educational experience for the faculty and the students.
- Nursing educators need to be aware of the role they play in reshaping health care and defining the discipline through theory development, testing, evaluation, and the educational process.
- Curriculum development that focuses on the contributions of the discipline to care outcomes places nursing knowledge as central to the teaching/ learning experience. Even when knowledge about physiologic stability is critical to the nurse's role, care of the whole human needs to remain the focus of the nurse–patient encounter.
- HEC helps nurses in all settings of professional practice give voice to what they know and helps them to articulate the differences in and contributions of nursing care to other providers.

A Force for Social Change

"Theory adequate to the task of changing the world must be open-ended, nondogmatic, informing and grounded in the circumstances of everyday life" (Lather, 1986, p. 262). HEC offers participants an opportunity to focus on pattern recognition in a unique way. The encounter alone can be life changing for all involved. Individuals need the knowledge and support of nurses to create movement, alleviate suffering, and create opportunities for individuals to recognize their potential.

HEC is person oriented. It goes to the individual experiencing a situation and offers time and knowledge to meet the person where he or she is and work in a mutual process to find new alternatives to relieve suffering, promote justice, and advance the common good for all. Thomas Moore expresses this best when he states "care of the soul . . . isn't about curing and fixing, changing adjusting or making healthy . . . It does not look to the future for an ideal . . . Rather it remains patiently in the present, close to life as it presents itself day by day" (1992, p. xv).

Final Thoughts

Nursing knowledge continues to grow through the development and testing of theory. Theory development at the midrange and practice levels can be used to bring nursing knowledge to the patient experience in unique ways. HEC is one theoretical perspective that appeals to nurse scholars because it is innovative, celebrates nursing as a discipline and a science, and can easily link knowledge to research and practice. HEC promotes the use of nursing knowledge and practice wisdom (Litchfield, 1999) to create an environment of care that acknowledges nursing's moral imperative to patients (Hayes, Chapter 4) and optimizes opportunities for expanding consciousness in nurses and patients, during health and illness.

References

Barron, A. M. (2000). Life meanings and the experience of cancer. *Dissertation Abstracts International*, 54 (UMI No. 30-08589).

Bentov, I. (1978). *Stalking the wild pendulum*. New York, NY: E. P. Dutton.

Berry, D. (2004). An emerging model of behavior change in women maintaining weight loss. *Nursing Science Quarterly*, 17(3), 242–245.

Bohm, D. (1980). *Wholeness and the implicate order*. London: Routledge & Kegan Paul.

Chinn, P. & Kramer, M. K. (1999). *Theory and nursing: Integrated knowledge development* (5th ed). St. Louis, MO: Mosby.

Consensus Document. (1998). In: Sr. Callista Roy & D. Jones, (Eds.). *Nursing knowledge development and clinical practice: Opportunities and direction*. New York, NY: Springer (in press).

Hayes, C. *Dissertation Abstracts International* Unpublished dissertation, Boston College, Chestnut Hill, MA.

Jones, D. (2000). Linking nursing language with knowledge development. In: Norma L. Chaska, (Ed.). *The nursing profession: Tomorrow and beyond*. (pp. 373–385). Thousand Oaks, CA: Sage Publications.

Litchfield, M. (1999). Practice wisdom. *Advances in Nursing Science*, 22(2), 62–73.

McEwen, M., & Willis, E. M. (2002). *Theoretical basis for nursing*. Philadelphia, PA: Lippincott Williams and Wilkins.

Moore, T. (1992). *Care of the soul*. New York, NY: Harper Collins.

Neill, J. (2002). Transcendence and transformation in the life patterns of women living with rheumatoid arthritis. *Advances in Nursing Science*, 24(4), 27–47.

Newman, M. (1994). *Health as expanding consciousness* (2nd ed.). New York, NY: National League for Nursing Press.

Newman, M. (2001). Tetra-dialogue among scholars: Theory of health as expanding consciousness. Jan. 25, 2001.

Newman, N. (2002). *http://www.healthasexpandingconsciousness.org.*

Noveletsky–Rosenthal, H. T. (1996). Pattern recognition in older adults living with chronic illness. *Dissertation Abstracts International*. Unpublished dissertation, Boston College, Chestnut Hill, MA.

Noveletsky-Rosenthal, & H. T. Solomon, K. (2001). Reflections on the use of Johns' model of structures reflection in nurse practitioner education. *International Journal for Human Caring*, 4(2), 21–26.

Pharris, M. D. (2002). Coming to know ourselves as community through a nursing partnership with adolescents convicted of murder. *Advances in Nursing Science*, 24(3), 21–42.

Picard, C. (2000). Pattern of expanding consciousness in middle life women: Creative movement and narrative modes of expression. *Nursing Science Quarterly*, 13(2), 150–158.

Picard, C., & Margolis, T. (2002). Praxis as a mirroring process: Teaching psychiatric nursing grounded in Newman's health as expanding consciousness. *Nursing Science Quarterly*, 15(2), 118–122.

Prigogine, I. (1976). Order through fluctuation: Self-organization and social system. In: E. Jantsch & C. H. Waddington (Eds.). *Evolution of consciousness* (pp. 99–133). Reading, MA: Addison Wesley.

Rogers, M. (1970). *An introduction to the theoretical basis of nursing*. Philadelphia, PA: F. A. Davis.

Ruka, S. (2003). *Dissertation Abstracts International*. Unpublished dissertation, Boston College, Chestnut Hill, MA.

Wheeler, C. E., & Chinn, P. L. (1984). *Peace and power: A handbook of feminist process*. Buffalo, NY: Margaret-Daughters.

Young, A. M. (1976). *The reflective universe: Evolution of consciousness*. San Francisco, CA: Robert Briggs.

INDEX

A

Adolescents, pattern recognition and, 86–88
American Association of Critical Care Nurses (AACN), Certification Corp., 33
American Association of Nurse Executives (AONE), 106
American Nurses Association (ANA)
  Code for Nurses with Interpretive Statements, 33–34
  Nursing Administration: Scope and Standards of Practice, 108
  Social Policy Statement, 27, 32, 36
Art
  See also Reflective art
  knowledge and, 215–216

B

Binding (time) stage, 12, 13
Bipolar disorder, affects on parents
  background information, 133–134
  conclusions, 140
  findings, 136–140
  HEC concepts, 134
  literature review, 134–135
  study design, 135–136

C

Care
  dialogue on, 205–212
  environment of, 54–55, 58, 96–98, 105–114
  synchronous, 102–103
  views toward patient and type of, given, 192–193

Note: f = figure
      t = table

Care model, for a nursing home, 100–102
Caring and health, role of, 6–8, 66
Caring consciousness, use of term, 7
Case management model, 19
Centering (space) stage, 12, 13
Choice (movement) stage, 12, 13
Clinical practice
  environment of care in, 105–114
  HEC future and, 225–226
  models, 20, 50–51
Code for Nurses with Interpretive Statements (ANA), 33–34
Community, 74
  HEC and, 83–93
  health barriers for females, 90–93
  pattern recognition process for adolescents, 86–88
  patterns, 88–90
  unity and praxis, 85
Community-Based Collaborative Action Research (CBCAR), 90
Community Center of Excellence in Women's Health (CCoEWH), 90, 92–93
Conceptual model, 109
Consciousness
  See also Health as expanding consciousness (HEC)
  dialogue on, 205–212
  stages of, 12–13
Creative movement
  art, reflective, 121–122
  conclusions, 130
  dance as a mode of expression, 120–121
  described, 121–122

findings, 123–129
HEC concepts, 119–120
research, 122–123
Culture, HEC and, 18–19

D

Dance as a mode of expression, 120–121
De-centering (boundarylessness) stage,
    12, 13
Dementia, nursing home patients with
    care model, 100–102
    comfort, promoting, 98–99
    environment of care, creating, 96–98
    family and, 97
    pattern recognition, 99–100
    statistics, 95
    synchronous care, 102–103
Disorganization and disruption, growth
    from, 15–16

E

Education. *See* Mirroring praxis; Sense
        patterns, students and
    HEC, 214–215
    HEC future and, 226
End-of-life care
    clinical practice applications, 50–51
    examples, 47–50
    findings, 46–47
    HEC concepts, 45
    professional narrative, 43–45
    research methodology, 45–46
Environment of care, 54–55, 58
    in clinical practice, 105–114
    in a nursing home, 96–98
Ethics/ethical issues
    *Code for Nurses with Interpretive
        Statements*, 33–34
    exemplar, 37–38
    HEC and, 30–31, 34–37
    praxis model of care and, 150
    principles, 28–30
    resolving, 34

F

Family
    dementia and, 97
    patterns, 17–18

Family health, nursing praxis and
    defined, 73–74
    example, 74–77
    methodology, 78–81
    outcome and conclusions, 81–82
    Females, health barriers for, 90–93
Framing development of effectiveness,
    182
Freedom, potential, 12, 13

H

Health as expanding consciousness
    (HEC)
    applications, 223–224
    bipolar disorder and affects on
        parents and, 134
    community and, 83–93
    concept of, 4–6, 11–13
    conclusions, 163
    creative movement and, 119–120
    culture and, 18–19
    end-of-life care and, 45
    environment of care, 54–55, 58,
        96–98, 105–114
    ethics and, 30–31, 34–37
    example, 66–68, 69–71
    future and, 224–227
    as a guide for creative practice, 23
    as a guide for education and
        curriculum development, 23–24
    as a methodology, 22–23
    models of, 19–20
    multiple sclerosis patients,
        recognizing patterns in, 154,
        161–162
    nursing education and, 20–21,
        214–215
    pattern movement, 68–69
    photographs, use of, 162–163
    praxis model of care and, 150
    professional identity and, 179–181
    reflective art and, 121–122
    research and, 222–223, 225
    sense patterns, students and,
        179–181
    theory and, 220–221
Health barriers for females, 90–93
Holistic care, 32–33

I

Intentionality, 65–66, 216
Interactive-integrative paradigm,
    189–190
Interdisciplinary teams (IDTs), 102

K

Knowledge, 6, 12, 66
    art and, 215–216
    links to practice and, 193–195

L

Licensed Nursing Assistants (LNAs), 101

M

Mirroring praxis
    campus environment, 175–176
    conclusions, 177–178
    description of, 170
    meaning and pattern, 173
    mindfulness and presence, 172–173
    pattern appreciation, 174–175
    pattern appreciation, client's, 176
    pattern appreciation, student's, 177
    philosophical and theoretical
        aspects, 171–172
    self exploration, 173–174
Models
    creating practice, creating, 108–109
    terms related to, 109
Movement strategies, 14
Multiple sclerosis patients, recognizing
    patterns in
    background information, 153
    description of disease and people
        with, 154–157
    HEC concepts, 154, 161–162
    life patterns, 157, 158
    stories of patients, 159–161
    underlying patterns, 157–158
Mutuality, 33, 66

N

Newman, Margaret A., 3–9, 11–16, 28, 30,
    33, 34, 35, 36, 38
    See also Health as expanding
        consciousness (HEC)
    discussion with, 205–212

Newman Group, 110–114
Nightingale, F., 32
Nurse administrators
    care environments and, 105–107
    challenges for, 107–108
    nursing theory and, 107
    practice models, creating, 108–109
    theory-based practice example,
        109–110
Nurse case managers (NCMs), 101
Nurses, benefits of partnerships with,
    16–17
Nurse work
    critical aspects of, 65–66
    example, 66–68, 69–71
Nursing, defined, 31–33
*Nursing Administration: Scope and Standards
    of Practice* (ANA), 108
Nursing education, HEC and, 20–21
Nursing homes
    See also Dementia, nursing home
        patients with
    care model for, 100–102
Nursing praxis. *See* Family health,
    nursing praxis and

O

Observation strategies, 14

P

Paradigmatic perspectives, 189–190
Parallel pattern framing, 182
Particulate-deterministic paradigm, 189
    Patient-nurse relationships,
        exemplars
    aftermath and discussion, 197–199
    description of, 187–189, 192, 193, 195,
        196, 197, 198–199
    linking knowledge and practice,
        193–195
    linking theory to practice, 190–191
    recommendations for education,
        199–201
    treating patient as you would want to
        be, 196–197
    views toward patient and type of
        care given, 192–193
Pattern movement, 68–69

Pattern recognition
  See also Multiple sclerosis patients,
    recognizing patterns in
  adolescents and, 86–88
  community, 88–90
  defined, 4–6
  dementia and, 99–100
  disorganization and disruption and,
    15–16
  partnership with nurses and, 16–17
  person-environment connection,
    14–15
  self, 18
  uncovering family, 17–18
Person
  American Nurses Association's view
    of, 27
  Newman's view of, 28
Philosophical framing, 182
Practice
  linking knowledge and, 193–195
  linking theory to, 190–191
Practice models
  creating, 108–109
  defined, 109
Praxis
  See also Family health, nursing praxis
    and; Mirroring praxis
  process, 8, 13–14, 75, 85
Praxis model of care
  assumptions, 143–144
  conclusions, 151
  ethical issues, 150
  findings, 149–150
  HEC links, 150
  hope/ideas actualization, 146–147
  practical applications, 147–148
  process, 144
  project team formation, 145–146
  proposal creation, 147
  proposal modification, 148–149
  research preparation, 145
Preadmission clinics (PACs)
  development of, 54–55
  environment of care, 54–55, 58
  implementation phase, 59–60
  practical applications, 57–58
  research findings and evaluation of
    nurses' experiences, 57

research findings and evaluation of
    patients' experiences, 55–57
  space for interviewing patients, 55
Preadmission Nursing Practice Model
    (PNPM)
  description and changes in, 54–55
  environment of care, 54–55, 58
  evaluation of, 61–62
  examples, 60–61
  purpose of, 53–54
Presencing, 66
Problem framing, 182
Professional identity, HEC and, 179–181
Professional practice model, 109

R
Reality framing, 182
Reflection
  as a process, 183–184
  structured, 181–183
Reflective art
  conclusions, 130
  described, 121–122
  findings, 123–129
  research, 122–123
Research, HEC and, 222–223, 225
Role framing, 182
Roy, Callista, 205–212

S
Sense patterns, students and
  curriculum integration, 185
  discussion and conclusions, 184–186
  HEC concepts and professional
    identity, 179–181
  reflection process, 183–184
  structured reflection, 181–183
Social change, 226–227
Social Policy Statement (ANA), 27, 32, 36
Structured reflection, 181–183
Students. *See* Mirroring praxis; Sense
    patterns, students and
Sunrise model, 8

T
Temporal framing, 182
Theoretical framing, 182
Theory
  HEC and, 220–221

linking practice and, 190–191
TheoryResearchPractice, 8–9

U
Unitary-transformative paradigm, 190
Unity paradigm, 85

V
Vision, 74

Visual representations, 14

W
Watson, Jean, 205–212

Y
Young, A. M., 12–13